HOMEMADE KOMBUCHA RECIPES

A Comprehensive Guide to Classic and Herbal Kombucha Recipes for Digestive Health and Immunity Boosting for Beginners & Seniors.

Daniel W. Lee

HOMEMADE KOMBUCHA RECIPES

TABLE OF CONTENT

CHAPTER ONE

INTRODUCTION TO KOMBUCHA

1.1 What is Kombucha?

Kombucha is a fermented tea beverage that has been enjoyed for centuries due to its unique taste and purported health benefits. Originating from East Asia, it has gained immense popularity worldwide in recent years, thanks to its refreshing flavor and probiotic content. But what exactly is Kombucha, and why has it captivated so many enthusiasts?

The Basics of Kombucha

At its core, Kombucha is a tea-based drink that undergoes fermentation with the help of a symbiotic culture of bacteria and yeast (SCOBY). This culture, often referred to as the "mother" or "mushroom" due to its appearance, transforms sweetened tea into a slightly effervescent, tangy, and often mildly alcoholic beverage.

Ingredients and Process

Tea: The base for Kombucha is typically black or green tea. These teas provide the necessary nutrients and tannins that feed the SCOBY and contribute to the final flavor profile of the drink.

Sugar: Sugar is an essential ingredient in the brewing process. It acts as food for the yeast in the SCOBY, which breaks it down during fermentation, producing alcohol and carbon dioxide. The bacteria then convert the alcohol into acetic acid, giving Kombucha its characteristic tang.

SCOBY: The SCOBY is a gelatinous mat that contains a complex ecosystem of beneficial bacteria and yeast. It is responsible for initiating and maintaining the fermentation process.

Water: Clean, filtered water is crucial for brewing Kombucha, as contaminants can interfere with fermentation and potentially harm the SCOBY.

The Fermentation Process

The fermentation of Kombucha occurs in two stages:

Primary Fermentation: This is the initial phase where sweetened tea is combined with the SCOBY and left to ferment for 7-14 days at room temperature. During this time, the yeast in the SCOBY consumes the sugar, producing alcohol and carbon dioxide. Concurrently, the bacteria convert the alcohol into acetic acid, creating the drink's signature sour taste.

HOMEMADE KOMBUCHA RECIPES

Secondary Fermentation: After the primary fermentation, the Kombucha can be bottled and sealed for a secondary fermentation. This stage, lasting 3-7 days, enhances carbonation and allows for flavoring with fruits, herbs, or spices. The sealed environment traps carbon dioxide, giving Kombucha its fizzy quality.

Taste and Varieties

Kombucha's flavor profile can range from mildly sweet to sharply tangy, depending on the length of fermentation and added flavorings. Common flavors include ginger, lemon, berry, and various herbal infusions. The balance of sweetness and acidity can be adjusted to suit personal preferences, making Kombucha a versatile beverage.

Nutritional and Health Aspects

Kombucha is praised for its potential health benefits, largely attributed to its probiotic content. Probiotics are beneficial bacteria that support gut health and digestion. Additionally, Kombucha contains antioxidants from the tea, vitamins, particularly B vitamins, and organic acids like acetic acid and gluconic acid, which have antimicrobial properties.

While scientific research on Kombucha's health benefits is still emerging, anecdotal evidence and traditional usage suggest it may aid digestion, boost the immune system, and provide detoxification benefits. However, it's important to consume Kombucha in moderation due to its acidity and potential alcohol content.

Historical Context

Kombucha's origins trace back over 2,000 years to ancient China, where it was known as the "Tea of Immortality." It spread to Japan, Russia, and eventually Europe, gaining popularity as a health tonic. The word "Kombucha" itself is believed to come from a Japanese term, although the drink is quite different from the Japanese Kombu tea made from kelp.

Modern Popularity

In recent decades, Kombucha has experienced a resurgence in popularity, particularly in the health and wellness communities. It's now widely available in stores, cafes, and restaurants, with a growing number of homebrewers crafting their own unique batches. The beverage has evolved from a niche health drink to a mainstream favorite, embraced for its refreshing taste and potential health benefits.

Kombucha is more than just a trendy beverage; it is a time-honored drink with a rich history and a promising future. Understanding what Kombucha is and how it's made can deepen your appreciation for this delightful and healthful beverage. Whether you're a beginner or a seasoned brewer, exploring the world of Kombucha offers endless opportunities for experimentation and enjoyment.

1.2 History and Origins

The history of Kombucha is as rich and effervescent as the drink itself, spanning over two millennia and traversing continents. Its journey from ancient times to modern-day popularity provides a fascinating glimpse into how a simple fermented tea has captivated and benefited various cultures.

Ancient Beginnings

China: The Birthplace of Kombucha The earliest known origins of Kombucha can be traced back to Northeast China (Manchuria) around 220 BCE, during the Qin Dynasty. It was revered as the "Tea of Immortality" due to its supposed health benefits. Legend has it that the Emperor Qin Shi Huang was among its early enthusiasts, seeking the elixir for its rejuvenating properties. This period marked the beginning of Kombucha's association with longevity and wellness.

Japan: Kombucha and Dr. Kombu Kombucha's journey continued to Japan in around 414 CE. The name "Kombucha" is believed to have originated from a Korean physician named Dr. Kombu, who introduced the tea to the Japanese Emperor Inkyo. The term "Kombucha" combines "Kombu" (the doctor's name) and "cha," the Japanese word for tea. In Japan, Kombucha was integrated into traditional medicine practices and appreciated for its health-enhancing attributes.

The Spread to Russia and Eastern Europe

Kombucha made its way to Russia and Eastern Europe through trade routes and cultural exchanges. By the early 20th century, it was widely consumed in Russia, where it was known as "tea kvass" or "grib" (meaning mushroom). Russian households commonly brewed Kombucha, valuing it for its refreshing taste and potential health benefits. The drink's popularity spread to other parts of Eastern Europe, including Poland, where it was also embraced as a home remedy.

Western Europe and the World Wars

During World War I and II, Kombucha's spread faced challenges due to the scarcity of tea and sugar. Despite these obstacles, the drink maintained a presence in Europe. In the 1960s, scientific interest in Kombucha surged in Germany, where researchers studied its microbial composition and potential health effects. This period marked the beginning of a more formalized understanding of Kombucha's fermentation process and its benefits.

The Modern Revival

1980s and 1990s: The Health Movement Kombucha experienced a resurgence in popularity in the West during the late 20th century, particularly in the 1980s and 1990s. The burgeoning health and wellness movement, which emphasized natural and fermented foods, played a significant role in this revival. Kombucha was rediscovered by health enthusiasts, who began brewing it at home and sharing their experiences within the wellness community.

2000s: Commercialization and Global Popularity The early 2000s saw the commercialization of Kombucha, with companies bottling and distributing it on a larger scale. This move made Kombucha more accessible to the general public and introduced a variety of flavors and brands to the market. The rise of health-conscious consumers and the growing interest in probiotic-rich foods further propelled Kombucha into mainstream popularity.

Present Day: A Global Phenomenon Today, Kombucha is a global phenomenon enjoyed by millions. It is widely available in supermarkets, cafes, and specialty health stores. The beverage has evolved beyond its traditional roots, with countless variations and flavor combinations catering to diverse tastes. Modern brewing techniques and innovative approaches have made Kombucha an integral part of the contemporary health and wellness landscape.

Cultural Significance

Throughout its history, Kombucha has held cultural significance in various societies. In China, it was linked to ancient medicinal practices and the pursuit of longevity. In Japan, it was integrated into traditional health regimens. In Russia and Eastern Europe, it became a staple of household remedies. Today, Kombucha symbolizes a fusion of tradition and modernity, bridging ancient wisdom with contemporary health trends.

The history and origins of Kombucha reflect a remarkable journey of cultural exchange, scientific discovery, and enduring appeal. From its ancient beginnings in China to its current status as a beloved global beverage, Kombucha's rich heritage underscores its timeless allure. Understanding this history not only enhances our appreciation for Kombucha but also connects us to a legacy of wellness that spans centuries and continents.

1.3 Health Benefits

Kombucha, a fermented tea, has gained widespread popularity not only for its unique flavor but also for its purported health benefits. While scientific research on Kombucha is still emerging, many of its health benefits are attributed to its probiotic content, antioxidants, and bioactive compounds. This section delves into the various health benefits of Kombucha, examining both traditional beliefs and contemporary scientific findings.

HOMEMADE KOMBUCHA RECIPES

Probiotics and Gut Health

Probiotics: Kombucha is rich in probiotics, which are beneficial bacteria that support gut health. These probiotics can help maintain a healthy balance of gut flora, which is crucial for digestion, nutrient absorption, and overall gut function. Regular consumption of probiotics has been associated with improved digestion, reduced inflammation, and a stronger immune system.

Digestive Health: The probiotics in Kombucha may aid in alleviating common digestive issues such as bloating, constipation, and irritable bowel syndrome (IBS). They help break down food more efficiently and promote the production of digestive enzymes, leading to better nutrient absorption and a more comfortable digestive process.

Detoxification

Detoxifying Agents: Kombucha contains glucuronic acid, a compound that plays a role in the body's detoxification process. Glucuronic acid binds to toxins in the liver, transforming them into water-soluble compounds that can be excreted through urine. This detoxification process helps the body eliminate harmful substances and supports liver health.

Antioxidants: Kombucha is also a source of antioxidants, particularly when made from green tea. Antioxidants combat oxidative stress and free radicals in the body, which can damage cells and contribute to aging and chronic diseases. Regular consumption of antioxidant-rich foods and beverages, like Kombucha, may help reduce the risk of chronic illnesses and improve overall health.

Immune Support

Immune-Boosting Properties: The probiotics and antioxidants in Kombucha contribute to its potential immune-boosting properties. A healthy gut microbiome, supported by probiotics, is closely linked to a strong immune system. Additionally, the antioxidants in Kombucha help protect the body's cells from damage, further supporting immune function.

Vitamins and Minerals: Kombucha contains various vitamins and minerals, including B vitamins (B1, B2, B6, and B12), vitamin C, and trace minerals such as zinc and iron. These nutrients are essential for maintaining a healthy immune system and supporting various bodily functions.

Mental Health and Mood

HOMEMADE KOMBUCHA RECIPES

Mood Enhancement: There is growing evidence that gut health is closely linked to mental health, often referred to as the "gut-brain axis." The probiotics in Kombucha may positively affect this connection by supporting a healthy gut microbiome, which in turn can influence mood and mental well-being. Some studies suggest that probiotics can help alleviate symptoms of anxiety, depression, and stress.

Energy Boost: Kombucha naturally contains small amounts of caffeine and B vitamins, which can provide a gentle energy boost. These components help improve mental alertness and reduce feelings of fatigue. Additionally, Kombucha contains organic acids that can help the body produce energy more efficiently.

Cardiovascular Health

Cholesterol and Blood Pressure: Some animal studies have shown that Kombucha can help lower cholesterol levels and regulate blood pressure. These effects are thought to be due to the presence of antioxidants and other bioactive compounds that support heart health. While more human studies are needed, these findings suggest that Kombucha may have a positive impact on cardiovascular health.

Blood Sugar Regulation: Kombucha has also been shown to help regulate blood sugar levels. This benefit is particularly important for individuals with diabetes or those at risk of developing the condition. The polyphenols in tea, combined with the fermentation process, may help improve insulin sensitivity and reduce blood sugar spikes.

Weight Management

Metabolism Boost: The combination of probiotics, organic acids, and polyphenols in Kombucha may help boost metabolism and support weight management. Probiotics can improve digestion and nutrient absorption, while organic acids like acetic acid have been shown to reduce fat accumulation.

Appetite Control: Drinking Kombucha may help control appetite and reduce cravings. The fermentation process produces compounds that can promote satiety, making it easier to maintain a healthy diet and avoid overeating.

Kombucha offers a range of potential health benefits, from supporting gut health and detoxification to boosting the immune system and enhancing mental well-being. While more scientific research is needed to fully understand and confirm these benefits, the existing evidence and anecdotal reports suggest that incorporating Kombucha into your diet can be a healthful and enjoyable practice. As with any health-related habit, it's important to consume Kombucha in moderation and pay attention to how your body responds.

1.4 The Basics of Fermentation

Fermentation is an ancient preservation method and culinary technique that transforms food and beverages through the action of microorganisms. The basics of fermentation involve the metabolism of sugars by bacteria, yeasts, or molds to produce various byproducts such as alcohol, acids, and gases. This process not only preserves food but also enhances its nutritional value and flavor. In the context of Kombucha, understanding the fundamentals of fermentation is key to successfully brewing this popular beverage.

What is Fermentation?

Fermentation is a metabolic process that converts carbohydrates (sugars) into alcohol or organic acids using microorganisms such as bacteria, yeasts, or molds under anaerobic (oxygen-free) conditions. The two primary types of fermentation relevant to Kombucha are alcoholic fermentation and acetic acid fermentation.

Alcoholic Fermentation: Involves the conversion of sugars into ethanol (alcohol) and carbon dioxide by yeasts. This process is central to brewing beer, making wine, and producing the initial stages of Kombucha fermentation.

Acetic Acid Fermentation: Involves the conversion of ethanol into acetic acid by acetic acid bacteria. This process gives Kombucha its characteristic tangy flavor and contributes to its preservation.

The Role of Microorganisms

Microorganisms are the driving force behind fermentation. In Kombucha, the primary microorganisms involved are:

Yeasts: These are responsible for converting sugars into alcohol and carbon dioxide during the initial stages of fermentation. Common yeasts found in Kombucha include Saccharomyces cerevisiae and Brettanomyces bruxellensis.

Bacteria: These convert the alcohol produced by the yeasts into acetic acid and other organic acids. The most important bacteria in Kombucha are Acetobacter xylinum and Gluconobacter species.

SCOBY: The symbiotic culture of bacteria and yeast (SCOBY) is a gelatinous mat that harbors these microorganisms. It initiates and sustains the fermentation process, ensuring the transformation of sweet tea into Kombucha.

The Fermentation Process in Kombucha

The fermentation of Kombucha involves two main stages: primary fermentation and secondary fermentation.

Primary Fermentation:

1. **Preparation of Sweet Tea:** The process begins by brewing tea (typically black or green tea) and dissolving sugar into it. The sweetened tea provides the necessary nutrients for the microorganisms.

2. **Inoculation with SCOBY:** The SCOBY is added to the cooled sweet tea, along with a small amount of previously fermented Kombucha (starter liquid) to lower the pH and kickstart the fermentation.

3. **Fermentation:** The mixture is left to ferment at room temperature for 7-14 days. During this period,

the yeast converts the sugar into alcohol and carbon dioxide, while the bacteria convert the alcohol into acetic acid and other organic acids. The result is a slightly effervescent, tangy beverage with a balanced flavor profile.

Secondary Fermentation:

1. **Bottling:** After the primary fermentation, the Kombucha is bottled and sealed. This stage often involves adding flavorings such as fruits, herbs, or spices.

2. **Carbonation:** The sealed bottles are left at room temperature for an additional 3-7 days. During this time, the remaining sugars are consumed by the yeast, producing carbon dioxide and enhancing the carbonation of the beverage.

3. **Refrigeration:** After the desired level of carbonation is achieved, the bottles are refrigerated to slow down fermentation and preserve the flavor.

Factors Influencing Fermentation

HOMEMADE KOMBUCHA RECIPES

Several factors can influence the fermentation process and the final quality of Kombucha:

Temperature: Fermentation typically occurs best at room temperature (68-78°F or 20-25°C). Lower temperatures can slow down the process, while higher temperatures can lead to over-fermentation and undesirable flavors.

Sugar and Tea Concentration: The amount of sugar and type of tea used can affect the fermentation rate and flavor. More sugar provides more food for the microorganisms, potentially resulting in a sweeter or more alcoholic Kombucha.

Fermentation Time: The length of fermentation impacts the taste and acidity of the Kombucha. Longer fermentation times generally lead to a tangier and more acidic beverage.

Oxygen Exposure: During primary fermentation, some oxygen exposure is beneficial for the growth of aerobic bacteria. However, excessive oxygen can lead to the growth of unwanted microorganisms.

Cleanliness: Maintaining a clean environment and sterilizing equipment is crucial to prevent contamination by harmful bacteria or molds.

The basics of fermentation provide a foundation for understanding how Kombucha is made and why it possesses its unique qualities. By leveraging the natural processes of yeast and bacterial metabolism, homebrewers can create a delicious, healthful beverage that has been enjoyed for centuries. Whether you're a novice or an experienced fermenter, mastering the principles of fermentation is key to producing high-quality Kombucha and exploring its diverse flavors.

1.5 Kombucha Culture and Community

Kombucha is more than just a fermented tea; it's a vibrant part of a growing culture and community. From ancient traditions to modern practices, the culture surrounding Kombucha encompasses a diverse array of enthusiasts, artisans, and health-conscious individuals. This chapter explores the rich culture and community that has blossomed around Kombucha, highlighting its historical roots, contemporary movements, and the social aspects that make it more than just a beverage.

HOMEMADE KOMBUCHA RECIPES

Historical Roots of Kombucha Culture

Ancient Traditions: Kombucha's roots can be traced back to ancient China, where it was revered as the "Tea of Immortality." Over centuries, it spread to Japan, Russia, and Eastern Europe, becoming an integral part of traditional health practices. Each culture developed its unique approach to brewing and consuming Kombucha, contributing to its rich heritage.

Folk Remedies and Home Brewing: Historically, Kombucha was often brewed at home and passed down through generations. Families and communities shared their SCOBYs and recipes, fostering a sense of connection and shared knowledge. This tradition of home brewing remains strong today, with many enthusiasts embracing the hands-on, artisanal process.

The Modern Kombucha Movement

Health and Wellness Trends: In recent decades, Kombucha has gained prominence in the health and wellness community. Its probiotic content, potential health benefits, and natural ingredients align with the growing demand for functional foods and beverages. Kombucha is now a staple in health food stores, cafes, and wellness centers, symbolizing a commitment to natural and holistic living.

Craft Kombucha Breweries: The rise of craft Kombucha breweries has mirrored the craft beer movement, emphasizing quality, creativity, and local production. These breweries often experiment with unique flavors, organic ingredients, and innovative brewing techniques, contributing to the diversity of Kombucha available on the market. Craft breweries also play a pivotal role in educating consumers about Kombucha and its benefits.

Sustainability and Ethical Practices: Many Kombucha producers prioritize sustainability and ethical practices, reflecting broader cultural values. This includes sourcing organic and fair-trade ingredients, using eco-friendly packaging, and minimizing waste. The Kombucha community often intersects with environmental activism, promoting a more sustainable and conscious way of living.

The Social Aspect of Kombucha

Sharing and Gifting: One of the hallmarks of Kombucha culture is the tradition of sharing SCOBYs and starter tea with friends, family, and fellow enthusiasts. This practice not only facilitates the spread of Kombucha brewing but also strengthens social bonds. Sharing a SCOBY can be a gesture of friendship, support, and community building.

Workshops and Classes: Kombucha workshops and classes have become popular, offering hands-on learning experiences for beginners and seasoned brewers alike. These events provide opportunities to learn about the fermentation process, troubleshoot common issues, and explore new recipes. They also serve as social gatherings where people can connect over their shared interest in Kombucha.

Online Communities: The digital age has fostered a thriving online Kombucha community. Social media platforms, forums, and blogs are filled with Kombucha enthusiasts sharing tips, recipes, and experiences. Online communities provide a space for beginners to seek advice, for experts to share their knowledge, and for everyone to celebrate their successes and troubleshoot challenges.

Festivals and Events: Kombucha festivals and events celebrate the drink and its culture. These gatherings feature tastings, workshops, and presentations by industry experts. They offer a chance for enthusiasts to explore different brands, discover new flavors, and immerse themselves in the world of Kombucha.

Kombucha as a Lifestyle

Daily Rituals: For many, drinking Kombucha is part of a daily wellness ritual. It's often enjoyed as a refreshing morning beverage, a midday pick-me-up, or a post-meal digestive aid. Incorporating Kombucha into daily life reflects a commitment to health and mindfulness.

DIY and Craftsmanship: Home brewing Kombucha is not just about making a drink; it's a craft that involves creativity, patience, and attention to detail. Many brewers take pride in their unique batches, experimenting with flavors and techniques. This DIY approach fosters a deeper connection to the beverage and a sense of accomplishment.

Culinary Uses: Beyond drinking, Kombucha is also used in cooking and baking. Its tangy flavor can enhance salad dressings, marinades, cocktails, and even desserts. Culinary experimentation with Kombucha is another facet of its versatile culture.

The culture and community surrounding Kombucha are rich and multifaceted, encompassing ancient traditions, modern health trends, and vibrant social interactions. From the communal sharing of SCOBYs to the rise of craft breweries and online communities, Kombucha has evolved into more than just a beverage—it's a lifestyle and a movement. Engaging with the Kombucha community offers opportunities for learning, connection, and a deeper appreciation of this remarkable drink. Whether you're a novice brewer or a seasoned enthusiast, being part of the Kombucha culture can enhance your experience and enjoyment of this ancient elixir.

CHAPTER TWO

GETTING STARTED

2.1 Essential Equipment

Embarking on your Kombucha brewing journey requires some essential equipment to ensure a successful and enjoyable experience. Having the right tools and supplies not only simplifies the process but also helps you produce a high-quality beverage. This chapter will guide you through the essential equipment needed to start brewing Kombucha at home, highlighting the importance of each item and providing tips on choosing the best options for your needs.

1. Brewing Vessel

HOMEMADE KOMBUCHA RECIPES

The brewing vessel is where the magic happens, providing a safe and stable environment for the fermentation process. The choice of the vessel can significantly impact the quality and safety of your Kombucha.

Material: The ideal brewing vessel is made of glass, as it is non-reactive and does not leach chemicals into the brew. Ceramic and stainless steel are also acceptable, but ensure that the ceramic is food-grade and free of lead-based glazes. Avoid plastic and metal containers, as they can react with the acidic Kombucha and release harmful substances.

Size: For beginners, a 1-gallon (4-liter) glass jar is a popular choice. This size is manageable and allows for enough Kombucha to enjoy and share. As you gain experience, you may opt for larger containers to produce more Kombucha in each batch.

Shape: A wide-mouth jar is preferable as it allows better airflow and makes it easier to add and remove the SCOBY. It also facilitates cleaning and monitoring the fermentation process.

2. SCOBY

The SCOBY (Symbiotic Culture of Bacteria and Yeast) is the heart of Kombucha brewing. This gelatinous, pancake-like biofilm contains the essential microorganisms that drive the fermentation process.

Source: You can obtain a SCOBY from a friend, purchase one from a reputable supplier, or grow your own from a bottle of raw, unflavored Kombucha. Ensure that the SCOBY is healthy and free from mold or discoloration.

Care: Store the SCOBY in a small amount of brewed Kombucha (starter liquid) and keep it at room temperature between batches. Avoid exposure to direct sunlight and extreme temperatures.

3. Starter Liquid

The starter liquid is the mature Kombucha from a previous batch, rich in acids and beneficial microorganisms. It helps to acidify the new batch, preventing the growth of harmful bacteria and kickstarting the fermentation process.

Quantity: For a 1-gallon batch, you typically need 1-2 cups of starter liquid. If you don't have enough, you can use store-bought raw Kombucha as a substitute.

Storage: Keep the starter liquid in a sealed container at room temperature or in the refrigerator if storing for an extended period.

4. Tea

Tea provides the nutrients necessary for the growth and activity of the SCOBY. The most commonly used teas are black and green teas, but other varieties can be used as well.

Type: Black tea is a classic choice due to its robust flavor and high nutrient content. Green tea offers a lighter flavor and additional health benefits. You can also experiment with white tea, oolong tea, or a blend of these. Avoid teas with added oils, flavors, or artificial ingredients, as they can harm the SCOBY.

Quantity: For a 1-gallon batch, use about 8-10 grams (roughly 4-5 tea bags) of tea.

5. Sugar

Sugar is the primary food source for the yeast in the SCOBY. It is essential for the fermentation process, as the yeast converts sugar into alcohol and carbon dioxide, which the bacteria then convert into acetic acid.

Type: Cane sugar is the most commonly used and reliable option. Other sugars like white granulated sugar, brown sugar, or raw sugar can also be used, but they may affect the flavor and fermentation speed. Avoid using honey, artificial sweeteners, or sugar substitutes, as they can disrupt the fermentation process.

Quantity: For a 1-gallon batch, use 1 cup of sugar.

6. Water

Water is a critical component of Kombucha, making up the majority of the brew. The quality of water used can significantly impact the taste and safety of your Kombucha.

Type: Use filtered or spring water to avoid contaminants and chemicals found in tap water, such as chlorine and chloramines, which can harm the SCOBY. If using tap water, let it sit for 24 hours to allow the chlorine to dissipate or use a water filter.

7. Cloth Cover and Rubber Band

A breathable cloth cover allows airflow while keeping dust, insects, and contaminants out of the brewing vessel.

Material: Use a tightly woven cloth, such as cotton, muslin, or a paper coffee filter. Avoid cheesecloth or other loosely woven fabrics that may allow particles to enter.

Attachment: Secure the cloth cover with a rubber band or string to ensure it stays in place throughout the fermentation process.

8. Measuring Tools

Accurate measurements are crucial for consistent results in Kombucha brewing.

Measuring Cups and Spoons: Use these to measure the sugar and starter liquid accurately.

Kitchen Scale: A kitchen scale can be helpful for measuring tea leaves or loose tea accurately.

9. pH Strips or Meter

Monitoring the pH level of your Kombucha ensures it is fermenting correctly and safely. Kombucha should have a pH level between 2.5 and 3.5.

pH Strips: Affordable and easy to use, pH strips give a quick reading of the acidity level.

pH Meter: A digital pH meter provides more precise readings but requires calibration and maintenance.

10. Bottles for Secondary Fermentation

Bottling your Kombucha for secondary fermentation allows for flavoring and carbonation.

Material: Glass bottles with airtight lids are the best choice. Swing-top bottles, also known as Grolsch-style bottles, are popular for their secure seal and ease of use. Avoid plastic bottles as they can leach chemicals and are prone to bursting under pressure.

Size: Choose bottles that are easy to handle and store. Standard sizes range from 12 ounces to 32 ounces.

Cleaning: Ensure the bottles are thoroughly cleaned and sterilized before use to prevent contamination.

Having the right equipment is essential for successful Kombucha brewing. By investing in quality tools and supplies, you can ensure a smooth and enjoyable brewing process, resulting in delicious and healthful Kombucha. As you become more experienced, you may expand your setup and experiment with different techniques and flavors. Remember, the key to great Kombucha is not just in the ingredients but also in the care and attention you give to the brewing process.

2.2 Ingredients Overview

Brewing Kombucha involves a few key ingredients that work together to create this fermented, tangy beverage. Understanding the role and importance of each ingredient will help you make informed choices and ensure successful fermentation. This section provides an in-depth look at the essential ingredients for Kombucha, their variations, and their impact on the final product.

1. Tea

Role in Kombucha: Tea is the foundation of Kombucha, providing the essential nutrients, flavor, and tannins needed for fermentation. The type of tea you choose can significantly influence the taste, color, and quality of your Kombucha.

Types of Tea:

- ✓ **Black Tea:** The most commonly used tea for Kombucha brewing, black tea provides a robust flavor and a rich color. It is high in tannins and nutrients that support the health of the SCOBY.

- ✓ **Green Tea:** Known for its lighter, more delicate flavor, green tea also contains antioxidants and nutrients beneficial for the SCOBY. Green tea Kombucha often has a lighter color and a slightly different taste profile compared to black tea Kombucha.

- ✓ **White Tea:** This tea is minimally processed and has a subtle, mild flavor. It is less common but can produce a delicate and smooth Kombucha.

- ✓ **Oolong Tea:** A partially fermented tea, oolong offers a balance between the strong flavor of black tea and the lightness of green tea. It can add a unique complexity to your Kombucha.

✓ **Herbal Tea:** While not true tea (as they are not made from the Camellia sinensis plant), herbal teas can be used in combination with traditional teas. However, they should not be used alone as they lack the necessary nutrients for the SCOBY. Herbal teas can add unique flavors and health benefits to Kombucha.

Tips for Choosing Tea:

✓ **Quality:** Use high-quality, organic tea whenever possible to avoid pesticides and artificial additives.

✓ **Purity:** Avoid teas with added flavors, oils, or artificial ingredients, as these can interfere with fermentation and harm the SCOBY.

2. Sugar

Role in Kombucha: Sugar is the primary food source for the yeast in the SCOBY. During fermentation, the yeast converts sugar into alcohol and carbon dioxide, which the bacteria then convert into acetic acid and other organic acids. This process reduces the sugar content and creates the characteristic tangy taste of Kombucha.

Types of Sugar:

HOMEMADE KOMBUCHA RECIPES

- ✓ **Cane Sugar:** The most common and reliable sugar for Kombucha brewing. It ferments consistently and produces a clean, balanced flavor.

- ✓ **White Granulated Sugar:** Similar to cane sugar, this is another widely used option for its consistency and neutrality.

- ✓ **Brown Sugar:** Contains molasses, which can add a richer flavor and color to your Kombucha. However, it may ferment more slowly and result in a different taste profile.

- ✓ **Raw Sugar:** Less processed than white sugar, it can be used but may also introduce impurities that could affect fermentation.

- ✓ **Alternative Sweeteners:** Honey, agave syrup, and other natural sweeteners can be used with caution. These may alter the flavor and fermentation process, and honey can have antibacterial properties that could harm the SCOBY.

Tips for Using Sugar:

✓ **Quantity:** For a 1-gallon batch of Kombucha, use about 1 cup of sugar. Adjusting the sugar content can affect the fermentation speed and flavor.

✓ **Dissolving:** Ensure the sugar is fully dissolved in the hot tea before adding the SCOBY and starter liquid.

3. Water

Role in Kombucha: Water makes up the majority of the Kombucha brew. The quality of the water used can significantly impact the taste and safety of the final product.

Types of Water:

✓ **Filtered Water:** Ideal for Kombucha brewing, filtered water removes chlorine, chloramines, and other impurities that can harm the SCOBY and affect fermentation.

- ✓ **Spring Water:** A good alternative, as it is usually free from contaminants and contains beneficial minerals.

- ✓ **Tap Water:** Can be used if filtered or left to sit for 24 hours to allow chlorine to dissipate. However, some municipalities use chloramines, which do not evaporate and require a filter to remove.

Tips for Using Water:

- ✓ **Purity:** Always use clean, filtered, or spring water to ensure the best results and avoid contamination.

- ✓ **Temperature:** Ensure the water is cooled to room temperature before adding the SCOBY and starter liquid to prevent killing the microorganisms.

4. SCOBY

Role in Kombucha: The SCOBY (Symbiotic Culture of Bacteria and Yeast) is the living culture that drives the fermentation process. It converts the sweet tea into Kombucha by producing acids, alcohol, and carbonation.

HOMEMADE KOMBUCHA RECIPES

Characteristics of a Healthy SCOBY:

- ✓ **Appearance:** A healthy SCOBY is typically opaque, light brown or beige, and has a gelatinous, rubbery texture. It may have brown stringy bits hanging from it (yeast) and can vary in thickness.

- ✓ **Growth:** During fermentation, the SCOBY will grow a new layer on top of the brew. This is a sign of active fermentation.

Tips for Maintaining a SCOBY:

- ✓ **Storage:** Keep the SCOBY in a small amount of starter liquid when not in use, and store it at room temperature in a clean container. Avoid exposure to direct sunlight and extreme temperatures.

- ✓ **Handling:** Always handle the SCOBY with clean hands and equipment to prevent contamination. Rinse your hands with vinegar before touching the SCOBY to avoid soap residue.

5. Starter Liquid

Role in Kombucha: The starter liquid is mature Kombucha from a previous batch. It helps to acidify the new batch, preventing the growth of harmful bacteria and initiating fermentation.

Source:

- ✓ **Previous Batch:** The best source of starter liquid is from a previous batch of Kombucha. This ensures it contains the necessary microorganisms.

- ✓ **Store-Bought:** If you don't have a previous batch, use store-bought raw, unflavored Kombucha as a substitute. Ensure it is unpasteurized and contains live cultures.

Tips for Using Starter Liquid:

- ✓ **Quantity:** Use 1-2 cups of starter liquid for a 1-gallon batch. This ensures the proper acidity and microbial content.

- ✓ **Storage:** Store the starter liquid in a sealed container at room temperature or in the refrigerator if keeping for an extended period.

6. Optional Ingredients for Flavoring

Role in Kombucha: Flavoring ingredients are typically added during the secondary fermentation to enhance the taste and introduce new flavors. This is an opportunity to get creative and personalize your Kombucha.

Common Flavoring Ingredients:

- ✓ **Fruits:** Fresh, frozen, or dried fruits such as berries, citrus, mango, and pineapple add natural sweetness and vibrant flavors.

- ✓ **Herbs and Spices:** Fresh herbs like mint, basil, and ginger, as well as spices like cinnamon, cloves, and vanilla, can add complexity and depth to the flavor.

- ✓ **Juices:** Natural fruit juices can be used for flavoring and adding sweetness. Ensure they are free from preservatives and additives.

Tips for Flavoring:

- ✓ **Quantity:** Add flavoring ingredients to taste, starting with small amounts and adjusting as needed. Typically, 1-2 tablespoons of fruit or juice per 16-ounce bottle is a good starting point.

✓ **Infusion Time:** Allow the flavored Kombucha to sit for 2-5 days during the secondary fermentation to develop the desired flavor and carbonation.

Understanding the essential ingredients for Kombucha brewing is crucial for achieving the best results. By selecting high-quality tea, sugar, water, and maintaining a healthy SCOBY and starter liquid, you can create delicious and healthful Kombucha. Experimenting with different flavoring ingredients during secondary fermentation allows you to personalize your brew and discover new taste sensations. With the right ingredients and a bit of patience, you can master the art of Kombucha brewing and enjoy this ancient, healthful beverage in the comfort of your home.

2.3 Choosing the Right Tea

Tea is the cornerstone of Kombucha brewing, providing essential nutrients, flavor, and tannins that nourish the SCOBY (Symbiotic Culture of Bacteria and Yeast) and contribute to the beverage's unique taste. Choosing the right tea is crucial for a successful brew and can significantly impact the flavor, color, and quality of your Kombucha. This section explores different types of tea, their characteristics, and tips for selecting the best tea for your brewing needs.

Understanding Tea Types

Tea comes from the Camellia sinensis plant, and the various types are a result of different processing methods. The main types of tea used in Kombucha brewing are black, green, white, and oolong tea. Each type offers distinct flavors and benefits.

1. Black Tea

Characteristics:

- ✓ **Flavor:** Black tea has a robust, full-bodied flavor with malty, fruity, or smoky notes.

- ✓ **Color:** It brews to a dark amber or reddish-brown color.

- ✓ **Nutrients:** High in tannins and antioxidants, which are beneficial for the SCOBY and the fermentation process.

Benefits for Kombucha:

- ✓ **Rich Flavor:** Provides a strong, traditional Kombucha flavor.

- ✓ **Nutrient-Rich:** Supports healthy SCOBY growth and fermentation.

Popular Varieties:

- ✓ **Assam:** Bold and malty, ideal for a strong brew.

- ✓ **Darjeeling:** Delicate and fruity, offering a more nuanced flavor.

- ✓ **Ceylon:** Balanced with bright, citrusy notes.

2. Green Tea

Characteristics:

- ✓ **Flavor:** Green tea has a lighter, more delicate flavor with grassy, vegetal, or floral notes.

- ✓ **Color:** It brews to a light green or yellow color.

HOMEMADE KOMBUCHA RECIPES

✓ **Nutrients:** Rich in catechins and antioxidants, which are beneficial for health and fermentation.

Benefits for Kombucha:

✓ **Delicate Flavor:** Produces a lighter, more refreshing Kombucha.

✓ **Health Benefits:** High in antioxidants, contributing to Kombucha's healthful properties.

Popular Varieties:

✓ **Sencha:** Fresh and grassy, a common choice for green tea Kombucha.

✓ **Matcha:** Powdered green tea with a rich, umami flavor (used in small amounts due to its intensity).

✓ **Dragonwell (Longjing):** Smooth and nutty, offering a mild flavor.

3. White Tea

Characteristics:

✓ **Flavor:** White tea has a subtle, mild flavor with sweet, floral, or fruity notes.

✓ **Color:** It brews to a pale yellow or light gold color.

✓ **Nutrients:** Contains lower levels of tannins but is rich in antioxidants.

Benefits for Kombucha:

✓ **Subtle Flavor:** Produces a gentle, delicate Kombucha.

✓ **High Antioxidants:** Contributes to health benefits without overpowering flavors.

Popular Varieties:

✓ **Silver Needle:** Delicate and sweet, with a light, refreshing taste.

✓ **White Peony (Bai Mudan):** Slightly stronger than Silver Needle, with fruity and floral notes.

4. Oolong Tea

Characteristics:

✓ **Flavor:** Oolong tea has a complex flavor profile, ranging from floral and fruity to toasty and nutty.

- ✓ **Color:** It brews to a light amber to dark brown color.

- ✓ **Nutrients:** Contains moderate levels of tannins and antioxidants.

Benefits for Kombucha:

- ✓ **Complex Flavor:** Adds depth and complexity to Kombucha.

- ✓ **Balanced Nutrients:** Supports fermentation and SCOBY health.

Popular Varieties:

- ✓ **Tie Guan Yin (Iron Goddess of Mercy):** Floral and creamy, with a smooth taste.

- ✓ **Da Hong Pao (Big Red Robe):** Rich and toasty, offering a robust flavor.

Tips for Choosing the Best Tea

1. Quality:

✓ Choose high-quality, loose-leaf tea whenever possible. It typically offers better flavor and nutrient content than tea bags.

✓ Organic tea is preferable to avoid pesticides and additives that could affect fermentation and health.

2. Purity:

✓ Avoid flavored teas (e.g., Earl Grey, chai) that contain oils, artificial flavors, or additives. These can interfere with the fermentation process and harm the SCOBY.

✓ Ensure the tea is free from any added ingredients that might disrupt the delicate balance of the Kombucha brew.

3. Blending Teas:

✓ Blending different types of tea can create unique flavor profiles and enhance the complexity of your Kombucha.

✓ A common blend is black and green tea, combining the robustness of black tea with the lightness of green tea.

4. Experimentation:

✓ Experiment with different types and blends of tea to discover your preferred flavor profile. Keep notes on the types of tea used and the resulting taste to refine your brewing process.

5. Consistency:

✓ Once you find a tea or blend that you like, stick with it for consistent results. Small variations in tea type and quality can lead to noticeable differences in your Kombucha.

Choosing the right tea is a crucial step in brewing delicious and healthful Kombucha. Each type of tea brings its unique characteristics and benefits to the brew, allowing for a wide range of flavors and styles. By selecting high-quality, pure teas and experimenting with different types and blends, you can tailor your Kombucha to your taste preferences and enjoy the full spectrum of flavors this ancient beverage has to offer. Whether you prefer the robust flavor of black tea, the delicate notes of green tea, or the complexity of oolong tea, the right tea choice will enhance your Kombucha brewing experience.

2.4 Understanding SCOBY

The SCOBY (Symbiotic Culture of Bacteria and Yeast) is the cornerstone of Kombucha brewing, playing a critical role in the fermentation process. Understanding what a SCOBY is, how it works, and how to care for it is essential for successful Kombucha brewing. This section delves into the characteristics, functions, and maintenance of the SCOBY, providing you with the knowledge needed to nurture and sustain this vital component of your Kombucha.

What is a SCOBY?

Definition:

✓ **SCOBY:** An acronym for Symbiotic Culture of Bacteria and Yeast, the SCOBY is a cellulose-based biofilm that houses the beneficial microorganisms responsible for fermenting sweet tea into Kombucha.

Appearance:

✓ **Structure:** The SCOBY resembles a gelatinous, rubbery disc, often light brown or beige in color. Its texture is smooth and slightly slippery, with a consistency similar to that of a thick jelly.

✓ **Layers:** As the SCOBY ferments the tea, it forms layers. Each batch of Kombucha will produce a new layer on the surface of the brew, indicating active fermentation.

Functions of the SCOBY

Fermentation:

✓ **Yeast:** The yeast in the SCOBY converts the sugar in the sweet tea into alcohol and carbon dioxide. This process creates the effervescence in Kombucha.

✓ **Bacteria:** The bacteria convert the alcohol produced by the yeast into acetic acid and other organic acids. This imparts the characteristic tangy flavor to Kombucha and creates a slightly acidic environment that inhibits the growth of harmful microorganisms.

Health Benefits:

✓ **Probiotics:** The SCOBY is a rich source of probiotics, beneficial bacteria that support gut health and overall well-being.

✓ **Detoxification:** The organic acids produced during fermentation can help detoxify the body by supporting liver function and aiding digestion.

Caring for Your SCOBY

Feeding the SCOBY:

✓ **Sweet Tea:** The primary food source for the SCOBY is sweet tea, made from tea (typically black or green) and sugar. This provides the necessary nutrients for the microorganisms to thrive.

- ✓ **Frequency:** The SCOBY should be fed fresh sweet tea every 7-30 days, depending on the temperature and brewing conditions.

Storage:

- ✓ **Between Batches:** When not actively brewing, the SCOBY can be stored in a small amount of mature Kombucha (starter liquid) at room temperature in a clean, covered container.

- ✓ **Refrigeration:** Avoid storing the SCOBY in the refrigerator, as the cold temperature can slow down or halt the activity of the microorganisms.

- ✓ **Long-Term Storage:** For extended breaks between brewing, the SCOBY can be kept in a "SCOBY hotel" – a jar with multiple SCOBYs submerged in Kombucha. This allows for easy storage and maintenance.

Handling:

- ✓ **Cleanliness:** Always handle the SCOBY with clean hands and use sterilized equipment to prevent contamination. Washing your hands with vinegar before touching the SCOBY can help avoid soap residue.

✓ **Exposure:** Keep the SCOBY away from direct sunlight and extreme temperatures. The ideal fermentation temperature range is between 68°F and 85°F (20°C to 29°C).

Health and Maintenance:

✓ **Observation:** Regularly check the SCOBY for signs of health. A healthy SCOBY is firm and uniform in color, with no signs of mold, which would appear as green, black, or white fuzzy spots.

✓ **Separation:** As new layers form, you can separate the SCOBY into individual layers to start new batches or share with other brewers.

✓ **Replacement:** Over time, the SCOBY may become too thick or dark, indicating it's time to replace it with a new, fresher layer.

HOMEMADE KOMBUCHA RECIPES

Troubleshooting Common SCOBY Issues

Mold:

- ✓ **Identification:** Mold appears as fuzzy spots in colors like green, black, or white. It grows on the surface and is easily distinguishable from the smooth, gelatinous texture of a healthy SCOBY.

- ✓ **Action:** If you detect mold, discard the entire batch, including the SCOBY, and start fresh with a new SCOBY and clean equipment.

Unusual Smell:

- ✓ **Normal Odor:** Kombucha should have a tangy, slightly vinegar-like smell. Any strong or unpleasant odors (e.g., rotten eggs) indicate something is wrong.

- ✓ **Action:** Investigate potential causes such as contamination, improper storage, or incorrect brewing conditions. Adjust as needed and consider starting a new batch with a healthy SCOBY.

HOMEMADE KOMBUCHA RECIPES

Slow Fermentation:

✓ **Causes:** Low temperatures, insufficient starter liquid, or an unhealthy SCOBY can slow down fermentation.

✓ **Solutions:** Ensure the brewing environment is warm enough, use enough starter liquid, and check the health of the SCOBY. If necessary, replace the SCOBY with a healthier one.

Overly Sour Kombucha:

✓ **Causes:** Extended fermentation time can result in overly acidic Kombucha.

✓ **Solutions:** Reduce the fermentation time or dilute the sour Kombucha with fresh sweet tea or water. Monitor the brewing process more closely to achieve the desired flavor profile.

Understanding and caring for the SCOBY is essential for successful Kombucha brewing. By recognizing the vital role the SCOBY plays in fermentation and maintaining its health, you can ensure consistent, high-quality Kombucha.

Proper feeding, storage, and handling practices, along with troubleshooting common issues, will help you nurture your SCOBY and enjoy the many benefits of this ancient, probiotic-rich beverage. With this knowledge, you are well-equipped to embark on your Kombucha brewing journey, creating delicious and healthful drinks at home.

2.5 Safety and Hygiene Tips

Maintaining safety and hygiene practices is crucial when brewing Kombucha at home to ensure the health and quality of your beverage. Proper hygiene not only protects your SCOBY from contamination but also prevents the growth of harmful bacteria and ensures a successful fermentation process. This section covers essential safety guidelines and hygiene tips to follow throughout your Kombucha brewing journey.

Safety Guidelines

1. Cleanliness:

- ✓ **Sanitize Equipment:** Before starting, clean all brewing equipment, including jars, utensils, and bottles, with hot water and soap. Rinse thoroughly to remove any soap residue.

✓ **Use Vinegar:** Wash your hands thoroughly with vinegar before handling the SCOBY or coming into contact with brewing equipment to avoid introducing harmful bacteria.

2. Quality Ingredients:

✓ **Use Filtered Water:** Ensure the water used for brewing is filtered or spring water to avoid chlorine and contaminants that can harm the SCOBY.

✓ **Choose Organic Ingredients:** Opt for organic tea and sugar to minimize exposure to pesticides and ensure a healthier fermentation process.

3. Proper Storage:

✓ **Room Temperature:** Maintain a consistent brewing temperature between 68°F and 85°F (20°C to 29°C) to support active fermentation. Avoid extreme temperature fluctuations.

HOMEMADE KOMBUCHA RECIPES

- ✓ **Away from Sunlight:** Store brewing vessels and SCOBYs away from direct sunlight to prevent UV damage and maintain the SCOBY's health.

Hygiene Tips

1. Handling SCOBY:

- ✓ **Clean Hands:** Always wash your hands thoroughly with vinegar before handling the SCOBY or reaching into the brewing vessel. Avoid using soap, as residues can harm the SCOBY.

2. Equipment Sanitation:

- ✓ **Regular Cleaning:** Clean brewing equipment after each use to prevent mold and bacteria buildup. Use hot water and soap, then rinse thoroughly.

- ✓ **Boiling Method:** Periodically boil glass jars and utensils to sterilize them completely. Allow them to cool before using them for brewing.

3. Airflow and Coverings:

- ✓ **Breathable Coverings:** Cover brewing vessels with tightly woven cloth or coffee filters secured with rubber bands to allow airflow while preventing dust and insects from entering.

✓ **Avoid Cheese Cloth:** Do not use cheesecloth or other loosely woven fabrics that may allow contaminants to enter the brew.

During Fermentation

1. Observation:

✓ **Monitor SCOBY Health:** Regularly inspect the SCOBY for signs of mold, which appears as fuzzy spots on its surface. If mold is detected, discard both the SCOBY and the batch.

2. pH Monitoring:

✓ **Use pH Strips:** Monitor the pH level of your Kombucha regularly using pH strips or a pH meter. The optimal pH range for Kombucha is between 2.5 and 3.5, indicating a properly fermented brew.

HOMEMADE KOMBUCHA RECIPES

Bottling and Storage

1. Sterilization:

- ✓ **Clean Bottles:** Thoroughly clean and sterilize glass bottles before bottling Kombucha for secondary fermentation. Boil bottles or wash them with hot water and soap, then rinse well.

2. Airtight Seals:

- ✓ **Secure Lids:** Use airtight lids on bottles during secondary fermentation to promote carbonation and prevent contamination.

3. Refrigeration:

- ✓ **Store in the Fridge:** Once Kombucha reaches the desired flavor and carbonation during secondary fermentation, store it in the refrigerator to slow down fermentation and maintain freshness.

HOMEMADE KOMBUCHA RECIPES

Troubleshooting

1. Unusual Smells or Tastes:

- ✓ **Check Ingredients:** Review the tea, sugar, and water quality. Ensure all ingredients are fresh and free from contaminants.

- ✓ **Sanitize Equipment:** If the batch develops off-putting odors or flavors, sanitize brewing equipment thoroughly before starting a new batch.

2. Mold or Contamination:

- ✓ **Immediate Action:** If mold is present on the SCOBY or in the batch, discard both the SCOBY and the brew immediately. Clean all equipment and start fresh with a new SCOBY and ingredients.

By following these safety and hygiene tips, you can create delicious and healthful Kombucha while minimizing the risks of contamination or spoilage. Proper sanitation practices, quality ingredients, and regular monitoring of fermentation ensure a successful brewing process and maintain the health of your SCOBY. With attention to detail and a commitment to cleanliness, you can enjoy the benefits of homemade Kombucha safely and confidently.

CHAPTER THREE

THE BREWING PROCESS

3.1 Step-by-Step Guide to Brewing Kombucha

Brewing Kombucha at home is a rewarding and relatively simple process, though it requires attention to detail and adherence to basic principles of fermentation. This step-by-step guide will walk you through the entire brewing process, from preparing the tea to bottling your finished Kombucha.

Equipment Needed

Before you begin, gather the following equipment:

1. **Large Pot or Kettle:** For boiling water and brewing tea.

2. **Glass Brewing Jar:** A 1-gallon glass jar is ideal for primary fermentation.

3. **Cloth Covering:** Tightly woven cloth or coffee filters to cover the jar.

4. **Rubber Band:** To secure the cloth covering.

5. **pH Strips or pH Meter:** For monitoring the acidity of your Kombucha.

6. **Glass Bottles:** For bottling the finished Kombucha after secondary fermentation.

7. **Funnel:** To aid in transferring Kombucha to bottles.

8. **Stainless Steel Spoon:** For stirring and handling the SCOBY.

9. **Clean Towels and Vinegar:** For cleaning and sanitizing surfaces and hands.

Ingredients

1. **Tea:** Choose high-quality tea, such as black, green, or a combination, based on your flavor preferences and the characteristics you want in your Kombucha.

2. **Sugar:** Use regular granulated sugar or organic cane sugar. Avoid honey or other alternative sweeteners for primary fermentation, as they can affect the SCOBY.

3. **SCOBY:** Obtain a healthy SCOBY from a reputable source or from a previous batch of Kombucha.

4. **Starter Liquid:** Matured Kombucha from a previous batch, which helps to lower the pH and prevent contamination.

Brewing Steps

Step 1: Prepare Your Brewing Environment

✓ **Cleanliness:** Ensure all equipment is thoroughly cleaned and sanitized to prevent contamination. Wash hands with vinegar to remove any residues that could harm the SCOBY.

Step 2: Brew the Tea

1. **Boil Water:** Bring 4 cups (1 liter) of water to a boil in a large pot or kettle.

2. **Steep Tea:** Remove the water from heat and add 4-6 teaspoons (20-30 grams) of loose tea or 4-6 tea bags. Steep for 10-15 minutes, depending on the type of tea and desired strength.

3. **Add Sugar:** Stir in 1 cup (200 grams) of sugar until completely dissolved. This provides the necessary food for the SCOBY.

Step 3: Cool the Sweet Tea Mixture

✓ **Room Temperature:** Allow the sweet tea mixture to cool to room temperature, approximately 68-85°F (20-29°C). Avoid adding the SCOBY to hot tea, as it can damage or kill the microorganisms.

Step 4: Combine Tea and SCOBY

1. **Transfer to Brewing Jar:** Pour the cooled sweet tea mixture into the glass brewing jar.

2. **Add Starter Liquid:** Pour in 1-2 cups (250-500 ml) of matured Kombucha from a previous batch. This lowers the pH and provides beneficial bacteria to kickstart fermentation.

3. **Place the SCOBY:** Gently slide the SCOBY into the jar, ensuring it floats on the surface of the tea. The smoother side of the SCOBY should face upward.

Step 5: Cover and Ferment

1. **Cover Securely:** Place a tightly woven cloth or coffee filter over the mouth of the jar. Secure with a rubber band to prevent dust, insects, and contaminants from entering.

HOMEMADE KOMBUCHA RECIPES

2. **Fermentation Time:** Store the jar in a warm, dark place away from direct sunlight. Allow the Kombucha to ferment undisturbed for 7-14 days, depending on temperature and desired taste. Warmer temperatures ferment faster than cooler ones.

Step 6: Monitor Fermentation

✓ **Observation:** Check the Kombucha periodically after 7 days. Taste a small amount using a clean spoon to determine if it has reached the desired flavor and acidity. The longer it ferments, the tangier it becomes.

Step 7: Bottle the Kombucha

1. **Prepare Bottles:** Wash and sanitize glass bottles and lids thoroughly. Boil them or use hot water and soap, then rinse well.

2. **Remove SCOBY:** Carefully remove the SCOBY and set it aside on a clean plate or bowl. Reserve 1-2 cups of the fermented Kombucha as starter liquid for your next batch.

3. **Flavoring (Optional):** Add fruit juice, herbs, or spices to the bottles for secondary fermentation and flavoring. Use a funnel to aid in pouring.

Step 8: Secondary Fermentation

1. **Seal Bottles:** Tightly seal the bottles with caps or lids to trap carbonation during secondary fermentation.

2. **Store:** Place the sealed bottles in a warm, dark place for 1-7 days to allow carbonation to develop. Check periodically by gently opening a bottle to release excess gas (burping).

Step 9: Refrigerate and Enjoy

✓ **Chill:** Once the Kombucha reaches the desired level of carbonation and flavor, refrigerate the bottles to slow down fermentation and maintain freshness.

✓ **Serve Cold:** Serve chilled Kombucha over ice, and enjoy its refreshing taste and health benefits.

Tips for Success

- ✓ **Consistency:** Maintain a consistent brewing environment and follow the same procedure for each batch to achieve consistent results.

- ✓ **Experiment:** Feel free to experiment with different tea blends, flavorings, and fermentation times to discover your favorite Kombucha variations.

- ✓ **Patience:** Brewing Kombucha requires patience, as fermentation times can vary based on temperature and other factors. Taste test regularly to achieve your desired flavor profile.

By following this step-by-step guide to brewing Kombucha, you can create delicious and healthful batches at home. From preparing the sweet tea mixture to fermenting with the SCOBY and bottling for secondary fermentation, each step is essential to producing high-quality Kombucha. With practice and attention to detail, you'll master the art of Kombucha brewing and enjoy the satisfaction of crafting your own probiotic-rich beverage.

3.2 Primary Fermentation

Primary fermentation is the initial stage of the Kombucha brewing process where the SCOBY (Symbiotic Culture of Bacteria and Yeast) transforms sweet tea into tart and effervescent Kombucha. This phase is crucial for establishing the foundation of flavor, acidity, and probiotic content in your brew. Here's an in-depth look at what happens during primary fermentation and how to manage this stage effectively.

What Happens During Primary Fermentation?

1. SCOBY Activity:

- ✓ **Yeast Action:** The yeast in the SCOBY consumes the sugars in the sweet tea, converting them into alcohol and carbon dioxide.

- ✓ **Bacterial Action:** Acetobacter bacteria in the SCOBY then convert the alcohol into acetic acid and other organic acids, giving Kombucha its characteristic tangy flavor.

2. Flavor Development:

- ✓ **Transformation:** Over time, the sweet tea mixture undergoes a transformation from a sugary solution to a tart and slightly acidic beverage.

- ✓ **Complexity:** The flavor profile develops complexity as various organic acids, enzymes, and aromatic compounds are produced during fermentation.

3. pH and Acidity:

- ✓ **pH Level:** The pH of the brew decreases as fermentation progresses, typically reaching a range of 2.5 to 3.5 by the end of primary fermentation.

- ✓ **Taste Testing:** Regularly taste the Kombucha during fermentation to monitor its acidity and determine when it has reached the desired balance of sweetness and tartness.

4. SCOBY Growth:

- ✓ **New Layers:** During fermentation, the SCOBY may grow a new layer on its surface. This is normal and indicates healthy fermentation activity.

✓ **Thickness:** The SCOBY may also thicken over time as it absorbs nutrients from the tea and produces new cellulose layers.

Managing Primary Fermentation

1. Temperature Control:

✓ **Ideal Range:** Maintain a consistent temperature between 68°F and 85°F (20°C to 29°C) throughout fermentation. Warmer temperatures accelerate fermentation, while cooler temperatures slow it down.

2. Fermentation Time:

✓ **Duration:** Primary fermentation typically lasts 7 to 14 days, depending on factors such as temperature, SCOBY health, and desired flavor intensity.

✓ **Taste Testing:** Begin tasting the Kombucha around day 7 to assess its flavor and acidity. Continue tasting every day or two until it reaches your preferred taste profile.

3. Observations:

- ✓ **SCOBY Health:** Regularly check the SCOBY for signs of health, such as a smooth surface and uniform color. Avoid disturbing the SCOBY unnecessarily to prevent contamination.

4. Covering and Airflow:

- ✓ **Breathable Cover:** Use a tightly woven cloth or coffee filter secured with a rubber band to cover the brewing jar. This allows airflow while preventing contaminants from entering.

5. pH Monitoring:

- ✓ **Testing pH:** Use pH strips or a pH meter to monitor the acidity of the Kombucha. The optimal pH range for finished Kombucha is typically between 2.5 and 3.5.

6. Starter Liquid:

✓ **Importance:** Ensure each batch of Kombucha includes sufficient starter liquid from a previous batch. This lowers the pH quickly and helps maintain a favorable environment for the SCOBY.

Signs of Successful Primary Fermentation

1. Acidity: The Kombucha develops a tangy, slightly vinegary taste that is characteristic of properly fermented brews.

2. Carbonation: During primary fermentation, some carbonation may develop naturally. This can vary depending on factors such as temperature and the amount of dissolved carbon dioxide.

3. SCOBY Health: The SCOBY remains healthy, with a smooth texture and uniform appearance. It may have grown a new layer during fermentation, indicating active fermentation.

Mastering primary fermentation is key to producing delicious and healthful Kombucha at home. By understanding the roles of the SCOBY, monitoring fermentation conditions, and tasting the brew regularly, you can achieve optimal flavor and acidity in your Kombucha.

This foundational stage sets the stage for secondary fermentation and flavoring, where you can further customize your brew to suit your taste preferences. With practice and attention to detail, you'll enjoy the satisfaction of brewing your own probiotic-rich Kombucha, ready to be enjoyed straight or flavored in endless creative ways.

3.3 Secondary Fermentation

Secondary fermentation is the phase of Kombucha brewing where the fermented tea undergoes additional carbonation and flavor development. This stage follows primary fermentation and allows you to enhance the taste, effervescence, and complexity of your Kombucha. Here's a detailed exploration of what happens during secondary fermentation and how to manage this crucial step in crafting your homemade Kombucha.

What Happens During Secondary Fermentation?

1. Carbonation Development:

- ✓ **Sealed Environment:** During secondary fermentation, the brewed Kombucha is transferred into sealed bottles or jars.

✓ **Remaining Sugars:** Any remaining sugars in the Kombucha can ferment further, producing carbon dioxide that becomes trapped in the sealed container.

✓ **Natural Carbonation:** This process naturally carbonates the Kombucha, resulting in a fizzy texture similar to commercial carbonated beverages.

2. Flavor Infusion:

✓ **Additives:** Optional ingredients such as fruit juices, herbs, spices, or ginger can be added to the bottles before sealing.

✓ **Flavor Extraction:** During secondary fermentation, these additions infuse their flavors into the Kombucha, creating a customized taste profile.

3. Enhanced Complexity:

✓ **Maturation:** The flavors continue to meld and develop over time as the Kombucha rests in a controlled environment.

✓ **Depth:** Secondary fermentation enhances the complexity of the brew, allowing for a richer sensory experience.

Managing Secondary Fermentation

1. Bottling Process:

✓ **Clean Bottles:** Ensure bottles are thoroughly cleaned and sanitized before transferring Kombucha into them.

✓ **Funnel Use:** Use a funnel to aid in pouring Kombucha into bottles, minimizing spillage and maintaining cleanliness.

✓ **Leave Space:** Leave a small amount of headspace (about 1 inch or 2-3 cm) at the top of each bottle to accommodate carbonation.

2. Adding Flavors (Optional):

✓ **Fruit Juices:** Add 1-2 tablespoons of fruit juice per 16 ounces (500 ml) of Kombucha to enhance flavor and sweetness.

✓ **Herbs and Spices:** Experiment with adding fresh or dried herbs, spices, or sliced ginger to create unique flavor combinations.

3. Sealing and Storage:

✓ **Tightly Seal:** Secure bottles with airtight lids or caps to trap carbonation during secondary fermentation.

✓ **Warm Environment:** Place the sealed bottles in a warm, dark place (similar to primary fermentation conditions) to facilitate carbonation and flavor infusion.

4. Fermentation Duration:

✓ **Timing:** Secondary fermentation typically lasts 1-7 days, depending on factors such as ambient temperature and desired carbonation level.

✓ **Monitoring Carbonation:** Check the bottles periodically by gently opening one to release excess gas (burping). This helps prevent over-carbonation and potential bottle explosions.

5. Refrigeration:

- ✓ **Chill Before Consumption:** Once the desired level of carbonation is achieved, transfer the bottles to the refrigerator to slow down fermentation and preserve freshness.

- ✓ **Serve Cold:** Serve chilled Kombucha directly from the refrigerator to enjoy its refreshing taste and effervescence.

Tips for Success

- ✓ **Consistency:** Maintain consistent brewing practices and conditions to achieve reliable results in carbonation and flavor development.

- ✓ **Taste Testing:** Sample Kombucha from one bottle during secondary fermentation to gauge its readiness. Adjust flavors or fermentation times in subsequent batches based on your preferences.

- ✓ **Experimentation:** Explore different flavors and ingredients to customize your Kombucha to suit your taste preferences and creative inspirations.

Secondary fermentation is an exciting stage in Kombucha brewing that allows you to refine the flavor, texture, and carbonation of your homemade brew. By understanding the principles of carbonation development, flavor infusion, and proper bottle handling, you can create effervescent and flavorful Kombucha tailored to your liking. With practice and experimentation, you'll discover endless possibilities for crafting delicious and healthful beverages that can rival any store-bought option. Enjoy the process and the satisfaction of sharing your homemade Kombucha with friends and family, knowing you've mastered this artful blend of science and creativity.

3.4 Bottling and Carbonation

Bottling and carbonation are crucial final steps in the Kombucha brewing process that enhance the flavor, texture, and overall experience of your homemade beverage. Proper bottling techniques ensure the preservation of carbonation while allowing you to experiment with flavors and achieve the desired effervescence. Here's a comprehensive guide on how to bottle your Kombucha and achieve optimal carbonation levels.

Bottling Process

HOMEMADE KOMBUCHA RECIPES

1. Prepare Clean Bottles:

- ✓ **Sanitization:** Thoroughly clean and sanitize glass bottles and their lids before use to prevent contamination and spoilage.

- ✓ **Boiling Method:** Boil bottles and lids for 10 minutes, or wash them with hot water and soap, then rinse well with clean water.

2. Remove SCOBY:

- ✓ **Gentle Handling:** Carefully remove the SCOBY from the brewed Kombucha using clean hands or utensils. Place it in a clean glass container with a small amount of Kombucha (starter liquid) for storage.

3. Reserve Starter Liquid:

- ✓ **Set Aside:** Reserve 1-2 cups (250-500 ml) of the fermented Kombucha as starter liquid for your next batch. This helps maintain the pH and supports the fermentation process.

4. Flavoring (Optional):

HOMEMADE KOMBUCHA RECIPES

✓ **Creative Options:** If desired, add flavorings such as fruit juices, herbs, spices, or sliced ginger directly to the bottles before filling with Kombucha. Use approximately 1-2 tablespoons of flavoring per 16 ounces (500 ml) of Kombucha.

5. Fill Bottles:

✓ **Using a Funnel:** Use a funnel to transfer the brewed Kombucha into the sanitized bottles. Leave about 1 inch (2-3 cm) of headspace at the top of each bottle to accommodate carbonation.

Carbonation Process

1. Seal Bottles Tightly:

✓ **Secure Lids:** Immediately seal each bottle with airtight caps or lids to trap carbon dioxide produced during secondary fermentation.

2. Secondary Fermentation:

✓ **Warm Environment:** Place the sealed bottles in a warm, dark place at room temperature (approximately 68°F to 85°F or 20°C to 29°C).

✓ **Duration:** Secondary fermentation typically lasts 1-7 days, depending on factors such as ambient temperature and desired carbonation level.

3. Monitor Carbonation:

✓ **Burping Bottles:** Periodically (every 24-48 hours), gently open one bottle to release excess gas (burping). This prevents over-pressurization and potential bottle explosions.

✓ **Visual Cues:** Watch for signs of carbonation, such as bubbles forming along the sides of the bottles or a slight hissing sound upon opening.

4. Refrigeration:

✓ **Chill Before Consumption:** Once the desired level of carbonation is achieved, transfer the bottles to the refrigerator to halt fermentation and preserve carbonation.

✓ **Serve Cold:** Serve chilled Kombucha directly from the refrigerator for a refreshing and effervescent beverage experience.

Tips for Achieving Optimal Carbonation

✓ **Consistency:** Maintain consistent brewing conditions and techniques to achieve reliable carbonation levels in your Kombucha.

✓ **Taste Testing:** Sample Kombucha from one bottle during secondary fermentation to gauge its carbonation and flavor. Adjust fermentation times or ingredients as needed for future batches.

✓ **Experimentation:** Explore different flavor combinations and ingredients to customize your Kombucha according to your preferences and creative inspirations.

Bottling and carbonation are essential final steps in the Kombucha brewing journey, enhancing the flavor, effervescence, and overall enjoyment of your homemade beverage. By following proper sanitization practices, carefully handling the SCOBY, and monitoring secondary fermentation, you can achieve optimal carbonation levels and create delicious, healthful Kombucha tailored to your taste preferences. With practice and attention to detail, you'll master the art of bottling and carbonation, delighting in the satisfaction of sharing your homemade Kombucha with friends and family.

3.5 Troubleshooting Common Issues

Despite following best practices, occasional challenges may arise during the Kombucha brewing process. Understanding how to identify and address common issues can help maintain the quality and success of your homemade Kombucha. Here are some troubleshooting tips for addressing common problems:

1. Unusual Odors or Off-Flavors

Issue: Your Kombucha has developed strange odors or flavors that are unpleasant or unexpected.

Possible Causes and Solutions:

- ✓ **Contaminated Equipment:** Ensure all brewing equipment is thoroughly cleaned and sanitized before each use. Use hot water and vinegar or a mild soap to clean equipment, rinse well, and avoid soap residue.

- ✓ **Quality of Ingredients:** Use fresh, high-quality tea and sugar. Ensure the water used is filtered or chlorine-free to prevent off-flavors.

- ✓ **Fermentation Temperature:** Maintain a consistent temperature range of 68°F to 85°F (20°C to 29°C). Extreme temperatures can stress the SCOBY and lead to off-flavors.

- ✓ **Fermentation Time:** Taste your Kombucha periodically during fermentation to monitor its progress. If it tastes overly sour or vinegary, it may have fermented too long.

2. Mold Growth on SCOBY

Issue: You notice mold growth on the surface of your SCOBY.

Possible Causes and Solutions:

- ✓ **Sanitation:** Ensure all equipment and hands are thoroughly cleaned and sanitized before handling the SCOBY. Use vinegar to clean hands and avoid soap residue, which can harm the SCOBY.

- ✓ **Airflow and Covering:** Use a tightly woven cloth or coffee filter secured with a rubber band to cover the brewing vessel. Avoid cheesecloth or loosely woven materials that may allow contaminants to enter.

✓ **SCOBY Health:** Monitor the SCOBY regularly for signs of mold. If mold develops, discard both the SCOBY and the entire batch of Kombucha. Start fresh with a new SCOBY and clean equipment.

3. Insufficient Carbonation

Issue: Your Kombucha lacks the desired level of carbonation, resulting in a flat beverage.

Possible Causes and Solutions:

✓ **Seal Tightness:** Ensure bottles are sealed tightly immediately after filling to trap carbon dioxide produced during secondary fermentation.

✓ **Secondary Fermentation Time:** Increase the duration of secondary fermentation to allow more time for carbonation to develop. Warmer temperatures generally facilitate faster carbonation.

✓ **Burping:** Periodically (every 24-48 hours), gently open one bottle to release excess gas (burping). This prevents over-pressurization and promotes carbonation in subsequent days.

- ✓ **Sugar Content:** Ensure there is sufficient residual sugar in the Kombucha before bottling. The yeast needs sugar to produce carbon dioxide during fermentation.

4. Slow or Stalled Fermentation

Issue: The fermentation process appears slow or has stalled, with minimal activity in the brew.

Possible Causes and Solutions:

- ✓ **Temperature Fluctuations:** Ensure a stable brewing environment within the temperature range of 68°F to 85°F (20°C to 29°C). Fluctuating temperatures can slow down fermentation.

- ✓ **SCOBY Health:** Check the health of your SCOBY. A healthy SCOBY should have a smooth texture and vibrant color. If it appears weak or thin, it may need revitalization or replacement.

- ✓ **Starter Liquid:** Ensure each batch of Kombucha includes sufficient starter liquid from a previous batch. Starter liquid helps lower the pH quickly and jumpstart fermentation.

✓ **Patience:** Fermentation times can vary based on factors such as temperature and SCOBY health. Allow sufficient time for fermentation to complete before making adjustments.

5. Over-Carbonation or Bottle Explosions

Issue: Bottles are over-carbonated or explode due to excessive pressure buildup.

Possible Causes and Solutions:

✓ **Burping:** Regularly (every 24-48 hours) open one bottle to release excess gas (burping) during secondary fermentation. This prevents over-pressurization and potential bottle explosions.

✓ **Bottle Quality:** Use sturdy glass bottles designed for brewing purposes. Avoid thin or weak glass bottles that may not withstand pressure.

✓ **Controlled Environment:** Store bottles in a warm, dark place during secondary fermentation, then refrigerate once desired carbonation is achieved to slow down fermentation and reduce pressure.

By troubleshooting common issues in Kombucha brewing, you can maintain the quality and consistency of your homemade brew. Regular monitoring, proper sanitation practices, and understanding the fermentation process are key to resolving challenges and enjoying delicious, healthful Kombucha. With patience and attention to detail, you'll refine your brewing techniques and confidently create batches of Kombucha that meet your taste preferences and expectations.

CHAPTER FOUR

FLAVORING YOUR KOMBUCHA

4.1 Introduction to Flavoring

Flavoring Kombucha is a delightful and creative process that allows you to customize your brew with a wide array of flavors, from fruity and floral notes to spicy and herbal undertones. Understanding how to effectively flavor your Kombucha opens up endless possibilities for creating unique and enjoyable beverages tailored to your taste preferences. This chapter explores the art and techniques of flavoring Kombucha, from selecting ingredients to balancing flavors and achieving consistency in each batch.

Why Flavor Your Kombucha?

1. Personalized Taste Profiles:

- ✓ **Variety:** Flavoring allows you to experiment with different combinations of fruits, herbs, spices, and other ingredients to create flavors that appeal to your palate.

- ✓ **Customization:** Tailor each batch of Kombucha to suit seasonal preferences or specific dietary needs, such as using organic ingredients or reducing sugar content.

2. Enhanced Enjoyment:

- ✓ **Appeal:** Flavoring enhances the sensory experience of drinking Kombucha, making it more enjoyable and refreshing.

- ✓ **Creativity:** Express your creativity by blending flavors and exploring new combinations that elevate the complexity and depth of your brew.

3. Health Benefits:

- ✓ **Nutritional Value:** Many flavoring ingredients, such as fruits and herbs, contribute additional vitamins, minerals, and antioxidants to the Kombucha.

- ✓ **Digestive Support:** Certain herbs and spices used in flavoring may offer digestive benefits, complementing the probiotic properties of Kombucha.

Selecting Flavoring Ingredients

1. Fruits:

- ✓ **Fresh or Frozen:** Use fresh fruits in season for optimal flavor, or frozen fruits for convenience and year-round availability.

- ✓ **Examples:** Berries (strawberries, raspberries, blueberries), citrus fruits (lemon, lime, orange), tropical fruits (pineapple, mango), stone fruits (peaches, cherries).

2. Herbs and Spices:

- ✓ **Fresh vs. Dried:** Fresh herbs provide vibrant flavors, while dried herbs offer concentrated aromatics and longer shelf life.

- ✓ **Examples:** Mint, basil, ginger, cinnamon, lavender, cardamom, cloves.

3. Floral Additions:

- ✓ **Edible Flowers:** Introduce delicate floral notes to your Kombucha for a fragrant and visually appealing beverage.

- ✓ **Examples:** Rose petals, hibiscus flowers, chamomile.

4. Other Additions:

- ✓ **Vegetables:** Experiment with vegetables like cucumber or beetroot for earthy or refreshing undertones.

✓ **Sweeteners:** Use alternative sweeteners like honey or maple syrup during flavoring for unique taste profiles.

Techniques for Flavoring

1. Primary Fermentation:

✓ **Direct Addition:** Add flavoring ingredients directly to the brewing vessel during primary fermentation. This allows the flavors to meld with the Kombucha as it ferments.

2. Secondary Fermentation:

✓ **Bottle Conditioning:** Add flavoring ingredients, such as fruit juices or herbs, directly to individual bottles during secondary fermentation. This method enhances carbonation and infuses flavors directly into the final beverage.

3. Cold Steeping:

✓ **Infusion:** Cold steep herbs, spices, or fruits in brewed and cooled Kombucha for 1-2 days in a sealed container in the refrigerator. Strain before consuming to remove solids.

4. Combination Approaches:

- ✓ **Layered Flavors:** Experiment with combining different flavoring techniques to create layered or complex flavor profiles. For example, use primary fermentation for fruit flavors and secondary fermentation for herbal infusions.

Balancing Flavors

1. Taste Testing:

- ✓ **Adjustments:** Regularly taste-test your flavored Kombucha during and after fermentation to monitor flavor intensity and balance.

- ✓ **Sweetness:** Consider the sweetness level of your Kombucha before and after flavoring. Some ingredients may require additional sweetening to balance tartness.

2. Consistency:

- ✓ **Record Keeping:** Keep notes on ingredient quantities and brewing times to replicate successful flavor combinations and achieve consistency in future batches.

- ✓ **Feedback:** Gather feedback from friends or family members to refine flavors and identify preferred combinations.

Safety and Best Practices

1. Sanitation:

- ✓ **Cleanliness:** Maintain strict sanitation practices when handling flavoring ingredients and equipment to prevent contamination and spoilage.

- ✓ **Tools:** Use clean utensils, bottles, and cutting surfaces to prepare and add flavoring ingredients.

2. Quality Ingredients:

- ✓ **Freshness:** Use fresh, high-quality ingredients to ensure optimal flavor and nutritional benefits in your flavored Kombucha.

- ✓ **Organic Options:** Choose organic ingredients whenever possible to minimize exposure to pesticides and chemicals.

Flavoring your Kombucha opens up a world of creative possibilities, allowing you to craft beverages that are not only delicious but also nutritious and tailored to your preferences. Whether you prefer fruity blends, herbal infusions, or exotic spices, understanding the principles of flavoring and applying best practices will help you achieve consistent and satisfying results with each batch. Embrace experimentation, keep detailed notes, and enjoy the journey of discovering new flavors and combinations that elevate your homemade Kombucha to new heights of taste and enjoyment.

4.2 Popular Fruits and Herbs

Flavoring Kombucha with fruits and herbs adds depth, complexity, and a burst of natural goodness to your brew. Here's a guide to popular fruits and herbs that you can use to infuse your Kombucha with delightful flavors:

Popular Fruits

1. Citrus Fruits:

- ✓ **Lemon:** Adds a bright, tangy flavor that complements the natural tartness of Kombucha.

- ✓ **Lime:** Offers a refreshing and slightly acidic twist to your brew.

- ✓ **Orange:** Provides a sweeter, citrusy profile with hints of zestiness.

2. Berries:

- ✓ **Strawberries:** Imparts a sweet, juicy flavor with a hint of tartness.

- ✓ **Raspberries:** Offers a bold, tangy taste that adds depth to the Kombucha.

- ✓ **Blueberries:** Provides a subtle sweetness and a rich, fruity aroma.

3. Tropical Fruits:

- ✓ **Pineapple:** Adds a tropical sweetness and a hint of acidity.

- ✓ **Mango:** Offers a sweet and aromatic flavor with a tropical flair.

- ✓ **Passion Fruit:** Provides a tangy and exotic taste that enhances the Kombucha's complexity.

4. Stone Fruits:

- ✓ **Peaches:** Imparts a delicate, fruity flavor with a hint of sweetness.

- ✓ **Cherries:** Offers a rich, slightly tart taste that pairs well with the Kombucha's acidity.

✓ **Plums:** Provides a subtle sweetness and a distinct fruity aroma.

Popular Herbs and Spices

1. Mint:

✓ **Peppermint:** Adds a refreshing and cooling sensation, perfect for summer brews.

✓ **Spearmint:** Offers a milder mint flavor with a hint of sweetness.

2. Ginger:

✓ **Fresh Ginger:** Provides a spicy and aromatic kick that complements the Kombucha's tanginess.

✓ **Crystallized Ginger:** Adds a sweet and spicy flavor with a chewy texture.

3. Floral Herbs:

✓ **Lavender:** Imparts a floral and soothing aroma, adding elegance to the Kombucha.

✓ **Rosemary:** Offers a pine-like flavor with a hint of herbal bitterness.

HOMEMADE KOMBUCHA RECIPES

4. Cinnamon:

- ✓ **Cinnamon Sticks:** Provides a warm, spicy flavor that pairs well with fruity or sweet Kombucha variations.

Tips for Using Fruits and Herbs

- ✓ **Freshness:** Use fresh, ripe fruits and herbs for optimal flavor and aroma.

- ✓ **Preparation:** Wash fruits thoroughly and remove any pits or seeds before adding to Kombucha.

- ✓ **Quantity:** Start with small amounts of fruit or herbs, then adjust according to taste preference in subsequent batches.

- ✓ **Infusion Time:** Allow fruits and herbs to steep in Kombucha during secondary fermentation for 1-3 days to extract flavors fully.

Flavor Combinations to Try

- ✓ **Citrus Mint:** Combine lemon or lime with fresh mint leaves for a refreshing and invigorating flavor.

- ✓ **Berry Blast:** Mix strawberries, raspberries, and blueberries for a vibrant and fruity Kombucha.

- ✓ **Tropical Paradise:** Blend pineapple and mango for a tropical escape in every sip.

- ✓ **Spiced Apple:** Add cinnamon sticks and a hint of nutmeg to apple-infused Kombucha for a cozy, autumn-inspired brew.

Experimenting with popular fruits and herbs allows you to create unique and flavorful Kombucha variations that cater to your taste preferences and seasonal inspirations. Whether you prefer the zesty tang of citrus fruits, the sweetness of berries, or the aromatic complexity of herbs and spices, understanding how different ingredients interact with Kombucha fermentation will help you craft batches that are both delicious and satisfying. Embrace creativity, keep notes on successful combinations, and enjoy the process of discovering new flavors that elevate your homemade Kombucha to a whole new level.

4.3 Spices and Roots

Enhancing your Kombucha with spices and roots introduces rich, earthy flavors and aromatic complexities that complement its tangy profile. Here's a guide to popular spices and roots that you can use to infuse your Kombucha with unique and satisfying tastes:

HOMEMADE KOMBUCHA RECIPES

Popular Spices

1. Ginger:

- ✓ **Fresh Ginger:** Adds a zesty and slightly spicy kick to your Kombucha, enhancing its natural tanginess.

- ✓ **Crystallized Ginger:** Offers a sweet and chewy texture with a spicy flavor that complements the brew.

2. Cinnamon:

- ✓ **Cinnamon Sticks:** Provides a warm, sweet-spicy aroma and flavor that pairs well with fruity or herbal Kombucha variations.

- ✓ **Ground Cinnamon:** Offers a concentrated cinnamon flavor that can be easily added to brewed Kombucha.

3. Cardamom:

- ✓ **Whole Cardamom Pods:** Imparts a complex, citrusy-spicy flavor with hints of herbal notes.

- ✓ **Ground Cardamom:** Adds a bold and aromatic profile, perfect for creating exotic Kombucha blends.

HOMEMADE KOMBUCHA RECIPES

4. Cloves:

- ✓ **Whole Cloves:** Offers a strong, pungent aroma and a warm, spicy-sweet taste to Kombucha.

- ✓ **Ground Cloves:** Provides a concentrated clove flavor that can be infused directly into the brew.

Popular Roots

1. Turmeric:

- ✓ **Fresh Turmeric Root:** Adds a vibrant golden hue and a mildly peppery, earthy flavor to Kombucha.

- ✓ **Ground Turmeric:** Provides a convenient way to add earthy and antioxidant-rich properties to your brew.

2. Licorice Root:

- ✓ **Dried Licorice Root:** Imparts a subtly sweet and herbal flavor with a hint of anise, enhancing the complexity of Kombucha.

- ✓ **Licorice Powder:** Offers a concentrated licorice flavor that can be easily infused into brewed Kombucha.

3. Dandelion Root:

- ✓ **Roasted Dandelion Root:** Adds a nutty and slightly bitter flavor profile that complements the natural acidity of Kombucha.

- ✓ **Raw Dandelion Root:** Provides a fresh and earthy taste, offering digestive benefits and richness to the brew.

Tips for Using Spices and Roots

- ✓ **Infusion Methods:** Add spices and roots directly to the Kombucha during primary or secondary fermentation to extract flavors fully.

- ✓ **Quantity:** Start with small amounts and gradually increase to achieve desired flavor intensity, as spices and roots can impart strong flavors.

- ✓ **Straining:** Consider straining brewed Kombucha to remove solids after infusion, especially for spices and roots that may leave residue.

Flavor Combinations to Try

HOMEMADE KOMBUCHA RECIPES

- ✓ **Ginger-Lemon Zest:** Combine fresh ginger with lemon zest for a zingy and refreshing Kombucha experience.

- ✓ **Turmeric-Citrus Blast:** Infuse Kombucha with fresh turmeric root and a blend of citrus fruits for a vibrant and healthful brew.

- ✓ **Cinnamon-Apple Spice:** Pair cinnamon sticks with apple slices for a warm, comforting Kombucha reminiscent of apple pie.

- ✓ **Cardamom-Orange Blossom:** Blend whole cardamom pods with orange peel for a fragrant and exotic twist to your brew.

Exploring spices and roots for flavoring Kombucha adds depth, character, and a unique twist to your homemade beverages. Whether you prefer the bold spiciness of ginger and cloves, the warmth of cinnamon, or the earthy richness of turmeric and licorice root, these ingredients offer endless possibilities for crafting flavorful and healthful Kombucha variations. Experiment with different combinations, adjust quantities to suit your taste preferences, and enjoy the creative journey of brewing and flavoring Kombucha at home.

4.4 Creative Flavor Combinations

Creating unique and delicious flavor combinations is a fun and rewarding aspect of brewing your own Kombucha. Here are some creative ideas to inspire your experimentation with flavors:

Fruity Combinations

1. Berry Blast:

- ✓ **Ingredients:** Mix raspberries, blueberries, and strawberries for a vibrant and antioxidant-rich blend.

- ✓ **Profile:** Offers a sweet-tart flavor with a refreshing fruity aroma.

2. Tropical Paradise:

- ✓ **Ingredients:** Combine pineapple and mango for a tropical escape in every sip.

- ✓ **Profile:** Provides a sweet and tangy flavor with a hint of tropical fruits.

3. Citrus Medley:

- ✓ **Ingredients:** Blend lemon, lime, and orange for a citrusy burst of flavor.

- ✓ **Profile:** Offers a zesty and refreshing taste with a balanced acidity.

Herbal and Spicy Combinations

1. Ginger-Lemon Zest:

- ✓ **Ingredients:** Pair fresh ginger with lemon zest for a zingy and invigorating Kombucha.

- ✓ **Profile:** Combines spicy notes from ginger with citrusy brightness from lemon zest.

2. Minty Fresh:

- ✓ **Ingredients:** Infuse Kombucha with fresh mint leaves and a hint of basil for a cool and herbaceous brew.

- ✓ **Profile:** Provides a refreshing and rejuvenating taste with a subtle minty aroma.

3. Spiced Apple Pie:

- ✓ **Ingredients:** Combine cinnamon sticks, apple slices, and a pinch of nutmeg for a comforting and aromatic Kombucha.

✓ **Profile:** Offers a warm, spiced flavor reminiscent of freshly baked apple pie.

Exotic and Floral Combinations

1. Lavender Lemonade:

✓ **Ingredients:** Infuse Kombucha with lavender buds and lemon slices for a floral and citrusy blend.

✓ **Profile:** Provides a delicate floral aroma with a refreshing lemony taste.

2. Hibiscus Spice:

✓ **Ingredients:** Blend hibiscus flowers with cloves and a touch of cinnamon for a rich and aromatic Kombucha.

✓ **Profile:** Offers a deep red color with a tart, floral, and spicy flavor profile.

3. Rosemary Citrus Twist:

✓ **Ingredients:** Combine rosemary sprigs with orange peel for a herbal and citrusy twist to your brew.

✓ **Profile:** Provides a fragrant herbal aroma with a hint of citrus freshness.

Tips for Creating Flavor Combinations

HOMEMADE KOMBUCHA RECIPES

- ✓ **Balance:** Aim for a balance of sweet, tart, and aromatic elements in your flavor combinations.

- ✓ **Experiment:** Start with small batches when experimenting with new flavors to gauge taste preferences.

- ✓ **Record Results:** Keep notes on successful combinations and adjustments made for future reference.

- ✓ **Seasonal Inspiration:** Use seasonal fruits and herbs for fresh and vibrant flavors that reflect the time of year.

The art of combining flavors in Kombucha brewing allows for endless creativity and personalization. Whether you prefer fruity blends, herbal infusions, spicy notes, or exotic floral aromas, exploring different combinations will help you discover unique and delightful Kombucha flavors. Embrace experimentation, trust your palate, and enjoy the process of crafting delicious and healthful beverages that cater to your taste preferences and creative inspirations. Cheers to brewing flavorful Kombucha that you and your friends and family will love!

4.5 Seasonal and Festive Recipes

Creating seasonal and festive Kombucha recipes allows you to celebrate flavors that are fresh, vibrant, and in harmony with the time of year. Here are some delightful recipes tailored to seasonal ingredients and occasions:

Spring Recipes

1. Strawberry Basil Bliss:

- ✓ **Ingredients:** Fresh strawberries, basil leaves.

- ✓ **Instructions:** Blend strawberries with a handful of basil leaves. Add to Kombucha during secondary fermentation for 1-3 days.

- ✓ **Profile:** Offers a sweet-tart strawberry flavor with herbal notes from basil, perfect for a refreshing springtime drink.

2. Lemon Verbena Delight:

- ✓ **Ingredients:** Lemon verbena leaves.

- ✓ **Instructions:** Steep lemon verbena leaves in brewed Kombucha during secondary fermentation for 1-2 days.

- ✓ **Profile:** Provides a citrusy and floral aroma with a lemony freshness, ideal for brightening up spring days.

Summer Recipes

1. Watermelon Mint Refresher:

- ✓ **Ingredients:** Fresh watermelon cubes, mint leaves.

- ✓ **Instructions:** Blend watermelon cubes with fresh mint leaves and add to Kombucha during secondary fermentation.

- ✓ **Profile:** Offers a juicy watermelon flavor with a cooling minty finish, perfect for hot summer days.

2. Pineapple Coconut Paradise:

- ✓ **Ingredients:** Pineapple chunks, coconut flakes.

- ✓ **Instructions:** Add pineapple chunks and a sprinkle of coconut flakes to Kombucha during secondary fermentation.

- ✓ **Profile:** Provides a tropical fusion of sweet pineapple and creamy coconut, transporting you to a beachside paradise.

HOMEMADE KOMBUCHA RECIPES

Fall Recipes

1. Spiced Apple Cider:

- ✓ **Ingredients:** Apple slices, cinnamon sticks, cloves.

- ✓ **Instructions:** Add apple slices, cinnamon sticks, and cloves to Kombucha during secondary fermentation for a warm and spicy infusion.

- ✓ **Profile:** Offers a comforting blend of apple sweetness with aromatic spices reminiscent of autumn.

2. Pumpkin Spice Latte Twist:

- ✓ **Ingredients:** Pumpkin puree, cinnamon, nutmeg.

- ✓ **Instructions:** Mix pumpkin puree with ground cinnamon and nutmeg. Add to brewed Kombucha during secondary fermentation.

- ✓ **Profile:** Provides a cozy and indulgent flavor with pumpkin spice notes, perfect for fall gatherings.

Winter Recipes

1. Cranberry Orange Cheer:

- ✓ **Ingredients:** Fresh cranberries, orange peel.

- ✓ **Instructions:** Combine fresh cranberries and orange peel. Add to Kombucha during secondary fermentation for a festive blend.

- ✓ **Profile:** Offers a tart cranberry flavor with citrusy brightness, evoking holiday cheer.

2. Peppermint Mocha Magic:

- ✓ **Ingredients:** Cacao nibs, peppermint extract.

- ✓ **Instructions:** Add cacao nibs and a few drops of peppermint extract to brewed Kombucha during secondary fermentation.

- ✓ **Profile:** Provides a rich chocolatey flavor with refreshing peppermint undertones, reminiscent of a holiday treat.

Tips for Seasonal Brewing

- ✓ **Freshness:** Use seasonal ingredients at their peak for optimal flavor and nutritional benefits.

- ✓ **Adjustments:** Taste-test your Kombucha during and after flavoring to adjust ingredient quantities for desired flavor intensity.

✓ **Presentation:** Garnish with fresh herbs, citrus twists, or seasonal fruits when serving for a festive and visually appealing presentation.

Seasonal and festive Kombucha recipes offer a delightful way to celebrate flavors that align with the time of year and special occasions. Whether you're enjoying a refreshing summer blend or a cozy winter infusion, these recipes provide creative inspiration to elevate your homemade Kombucha experience. Embrace the flavors of each season, experiment with ingredients, and share these flavorful brews with friends and family for memorable moments throughout the year. Cheers to brewing and enjoying delicious seasonal Kombucha recipes!

CHAPTER FIVE

RECIPES FOR BEGINNERS

5.1 Classic Kombucha

Making classic Kombucha at home is a straightforward process that yields a refreshing and tangy beverage. This recipe is perfect for beginners looking to master the basics of brewing Kombucha. Here's a step-by-step guide:

Ingredients:

- ✓ **Filtered Water:** 1 gallon (about 4 liters)

- ✓ **Granulated Sugar:** 1 cup

- ✓ **Black Tea Bags:** 4-6 bags (or 2-3 tablespoons loose black tea)

- ✓ **Kombucha Starter Liquid:** 1-2 cups (from a previous batch or store-bought)

- ✓ **SCOBY (Symbiotic Culture of Bacteria and Yeast):** 1 piece

Equipment Needed:

- ✓ **Large Pot:** For boiling water and steeping tea.

- ✓ **Glass Jar or Brewing Vessel:** 1-gallon capacity or larger, preferably glass.

- ✓ **Cloth Cover:** Breathable cloth (cheesecloth, paper towel, or clean cloth) secured with a rubber band.

- ✓ **pH Strips or pH Meter:** To monitor acidity levels during fermentation.

- ✓ **Bottles:** For bottling finished Kombucha (swing-top bottles are ideal).

Instructions:

1. Prepare the Sweet Tea Base:

- ✓ Boil 4 cups of water in a large pot.

- ✓ Remove from heat and stir in 1 cup of granulated sugar until dissolved.

- ✓ Add 4-6 black tea bags (or 2-3 tablespoons loose tea) and steep for 10-15 minutes.

- ✓ Remove the tea bags or strain loose tea and let the sweet tea mixture cool to room temperature.

2. Combine with Starter Liquid:

- ✓ Pour the cooled sweet tea into a clean glass jar or brewing vessel.

HOMEMADE KOMBUCHA RECIPES

- ✓ Add 1-2 cups of Kombucha starter liquid from a previous batch or store-bought Kombucha. This helps lower the pH and jumpstarts fermentation.

- ✓ Gently place the SCOBY on top of the sweet tea mixture, smooth side up.

3. Fermentation:

- ✓ Cover the jar with a breathable cloth secured with a rubber band to keep out insects and dust while allowing airflow.

- ✓ Place the jar in a warm, dark place (ideally 68-85°F or 20-29°C) to ferment for 7-14 days.

- ✓ Monitor the fermentation process by tasting the Kombucha after 7 days. It should taste slightly tangy and slightly sweet.

4. Bottling:

- ✓ Once the Kombucha reaches your desired level of tartness, carefully remove the SCOBY and set it aside.

- ✓ Prepare your bottles by washing them thoroughly with hot water and soap, then rinsing well.

HOMEMADE KOMBUCHA RECIPES

- ✓ Optionally, add flavorings like fruit juices, herbs, or spices to the bottles before filling with Kombucha.

5. Second Fermentation:

- ✓ Pour the fermented Kombucha into bottles, leaving a few inches of headspace at the top.

- ✓ Seal the bottles tightly with caps or lids and place them in a warm, dark place for 1-3 days to carbonate (secondary fermentation).

- ✓ Burp the bottles daily by gently opening them to release excess carbonation and prevent bursting.

6. Enjoy:

- ✓ After secondary fermentation, refrigerate the bottles to slow down carbonation and chill the Kombucha.

- ✓ Serve cold over ice, garnished with fruits or herbs if desired.

Tips for Success:

- ✓ **Sanitation:** Ensure all equipment and utensils are clean and sanitized to prevent contamination.

- ✓ **Temperature Control:** Maintain a stable fermentation temperature for consistent results.

HOMEMADE KOMBUCHA RECIPES

- ✓ **Patience:** Allow the SCOBY enough time to ferment the tea properly, adjusting fermentation time based on taste preferences.

- ✓ **Experimentation:** Once comfortable with the basic recipe, explore different teas, sweeteners, and flavorings to create your own unique Kombucha variations.

Troubleshooting:

- ✓ **Mold:** If you see mold on the SCOBY or surface of the Kombucha, discard the batch and start over with a new SCOBY and clean equipment.

- ✓ **Weak Fermentation:** Ensure the environment is warm enough and consider adding more starter liquid or sugar to kick-start fermentation.

Brewing classic Kombucha at home is a rewarding experience that allows you to enjoy a healthful, probiotic-rich beverage tailored to your taste preferences. With practice, you'll master the art of fermenting tea and confidently experiment with different flavors and techniques. Start with this basic recipe, refine your brewing skills, and soon you'll be sharing delicious homemade

Kombucha with friends and family. Cheers to your Kombucha brewing journey!

5.2 Ginger-Lemon Kombucha

Ginger-Lemon Kombucha combines the zesty brightness of lemon with the spicy warmth of ginger, creating a refreshing and invigorating brew. Here's a beginner-friendly recipe to guide you through making this delicious variation of Kombucha:

Ingredients:

- ✓ **Filtered Water:** 1 gallon (about 4 liters)

- ✓ **Granulated Sugar:** 1 cup

- ✓ **Black Tea Bags:** 4-6 bags (or 2-3 tablespoons loose black tea)

- ✓ **Fresh Ginger Root:** 1-2 inches, peeled and thinly sliced

- ✓ **Lemons:** 2-3, juiced (reserve some zest for optional garnish)

- ✓ **Kombucha Starter Liquid:** 1-2 cups (from a previous batch or store-bought)

HOMEMADE KOMBUCHA RECIPES

- ✓ **SCOBY (Symbiotic Culture of Bacteria and Yeast):** 1 piece

Equipment Needed:

- ✓ **Large Pot:** For boiling water and steeping tea.

- ✓ **Glass Jar or Brewing Vessel:** 1-gallon capacity or larger, preferably glass.

- ✓ **Cloth Cover:** Breathable cloth (cheesecloth, paper towel, or clean cloth) secured with a rubber band.

- ✓ **pH Strips or pH Meter:** To monitor acidity levels during fermentation.

- ✓ **Bottles:** For bottling finished Kombucha (swing-top bottles are ideal).

Instructions:

1. Prepare the Sweet Tea Base:

- ✓ Boil 4 cups of water in a large pot.

- ✓ Remove from heat and stir in 1 cup of granulated sugar until dissolved.

- ✓ Add 4-6 black tea bags (or 2-3 tablespoons loose tea) and steep for 10-15 minutes.

- ✓ Remove the tea bags or strain loose tea and let the sweet tea mixture cool to room temperature.

2. Add Flavorings:

- ✓ Add thinly sliced fresh ginger root directly into the cooled sweet tea mixture.

- ✓ Stir in the freshly squeezed lemon juice. Optionally, reserve some lemon zest for garnish after fermentation.

3. Combine with Starter Liquid:

- ✓ Pour the flavored sweet tea into a clean glass jar or brewing vessel.

- ✓ Add 1-2 cups of Kombucha starter liquid from a previous batch or store-bought Kombucha.

4. Fermentation:

- ✓ Gently place the SCOBY on top of the flavored tea mixture, smooth side up.

- ✓ Cover the jar with a breathable cloth secured with a rubber band to allow airflow while keeping out insects and dust.

✓ Place the jar in a warm, dark place (ideally 68-85°F or 20-29°C) to ferment for 7-14 days.

✓ Taste-test the Kombucha after 7 days to monitor its flavor development. It should be slightly tangy with a balanced ginger-lemon profile.

5. Bottling:

✓ Once the Kombucha reaches your desired level of tartness, carefully remove the SCOBY and set it aside in a clean container with some Kombucha starter liquid.

✓ Prepare your bottles by washing them thoroughly with hot water and soap, then rinsing well.

✓ Optionally, strain out the ginger slices and any sediment before bottling.

6. Second Fermentation (Optional):

✓ Pour the fermented Kombucha into bottles, leaving a few inches of headspace at the top.

✓ Seal the bottles tightly with caps or lids and place them in a warm, dark place for 1-3 days for secondary fermentation.

✓ Burp the bottles daily by gently opening them to release excess carbonation and prevent bursting.

7. Enjoy:

✓ After secondary fermentation (if performed), refrigerate the bottles to slow down carbonation and chill the Kombucha.

✓ Serve cold over ice, garnished with lemon zest if desired, and enjoy the refreshing flavors of ginger and lemon in your homemade Kombucha.

Tips for Success:

✓ **Fresh Ingredients:** Use fresh ginger root and lemons for vibrant flavors.

✓ **Taste Testing:** Adjust the amount of ginger and lemon juice based on personal preference and taste preferences.

✓ **Consistency:** Maintain a stable fermentation environment and follow sanitary practices to ensure successful brewing.

Troubleshooting:

✓ **Carbonation Levels:** If your Kombucha is under-carbonated, extend the secondary fermentation period or add a small amount of sugar before bottling.

✓ **Flavor Intensity:** If the ginger and lemon flavors are too strong, reduce the amount used in future batches.

Ginger-Lemon Kombucha is a delightful variation that combines spicy warmth with citrusy brightness, offering a refreshing and healthful beverage option. This recipe provides a simple and rewarding introduction to flavoring Kombucha at home. With practice, you can customize the ingredients and proportions to create your own signature blends. Enjoy the process of brewing and savoring your homemade Ginger-Lemon Kombucha, sharing its refreshing benefits with friends and family.

5.3 Berry Bliss Kombucha

Berry Bliss Kombucha infuses the tangy sweetness of berries into your homemade brew, creating a vibrant and antioxidant-rich beverage. Here's a beginner-friendly recipe to guide you through making this delicious variation of Kombucha:

HOMEMADE KOMBUCHA RECIPES

Ingredients:

- ✓ **Filtered Water:** 1 gallon (about 4 liters)

- ✓ **Granulated Sugar:** 1 cup

- ✓ **Black Tea Bags:** 4-6 bags (or 2-3 tablespoons loose black tea)

- ✓ **Mixed Berries:** 1 cup (such as strawberries, raspberries, and blueberries)

- ✓ **Kombucha Starter Liquid:** 1-2 cups (from a previous batch or store-bought)

- ✓ **SCOBY (Symbiotic Culture of Bacteria and Yeast):** 1 piece

Equipment Needed:

- ✓ **Large Pot:** For boiling water and steeping tea.

- ✓ **Glass Jar or Brewing Vessel:** 1-gallon capacity or larger, preferably glass.

- ✓ **Cloth Cover:** Breathable cloth (cheesecloth, paper towel, or clean cloth) secured with a rubber band.

- ✓ **pH Strips or pH Meter:** To monitor acidity levels during fermentation.

HOMEMADE KOMBUCHA RECIPES

✓ **Bottles:** For bottling finished Kombucha (swing-top bottles are ideal).

Instructions:

1. Prepare the Sweet Tea Base:

✓ Boil 4 cups of water in a large pot.

✓ Remove from heat and stir in 1 cup of granulated sugar until dissolved.

✓ Add 4-6 black tea bags (or 2-3 tablespoons loose tea) and steep for 10-15 minutes.

✓ Remove the tea bags or strain loose tea and let the sweet tea mixture cool to room temperature.

2. Add Mixed Berries:

✓ Rinse the mixed berries (strawberries, raspberries, blueberries) thoroughly under cold water.

✓ Optionally, cut larger berries like strawberries into smaller pieces.

✓ Add the mixed berries to the cooled sweet tea mixture.

3. Combine with Starter Liquid:

- ✓ Pour the berry-infused sweet tea into a clean glass jar or brewing vessel.

- ✓ Add 1-2 cups of Kombucha starter liquid from a previous batch or store-bought Kombucha.

4. Fermentation:

- ✓ Gently place the SCOBY on top of the berry-infused tea mixture, smooth side up.

- ✓ Cover the jar with a breathable cloth secured with a rubber band to allow airflow while keeping out insects and dust.

- ✓ Place the jar in a warm, dark place (ideally 68-85°F or 20-29°C) to ferment for 7-14 days.

- ✓ Taste-test the Kombucha after 7 days to monitor its flavor development. It should be slightly tangy with a balanced berry sweetness.

5. Bottling:

- ✓ Once the Kombucha reaches your desired level of tartness, carefully remove the SCOBY and set it aside in a clean container with some Kombucha starter liquid.

✓ Prepare your bottles by washing them thoroughly with hot water and soap, then rinsing well.

✓ Optionally, strain out the berries and any sediment before bottling.

6. Second Fermentation (Optional):

✓ Pour the fermented Kombucha into bottles, leaving a few inches of headspace at the top.

✓ Seal the bottles tightly with caps or lids and place them in a warm, dark place for 1-3 days for secondary fermentation.

✓ Burp the bottles daily by gently opening them to release excess carbonation and prevent bursting.

7. Enjoy:

✓ After secondary fermentation (if performed), refrigerate the bottles to slow down carbonation and chill the Kombucha.

✓ Serve cold over ice, garnished with fresh berries if desired, and savor the delicious berry flavors in your homemade Berry Bliss Kombucha.

HOMEMADE KOMBUCHA RECIPES

Tips for Success:

- ✓ **Fresh Berries:** Use fresh, ripe berries for vibrant flavors and nutritional benefits.

- ✓ **Adjustments:** Taste-test during fermentation and adjust sweetness or tartness by adding more or fewer berries.

- ✓ **Consistency:** Maintain a stable fermentation environment and follow sanitary practices to ensure successful brewing.

Troubleshooting:

- ✓ **Fermentation Time:** If the Kombucha is not tart enough after 7 days, allow it to ferment longer, tasting every few days until desired acidity is reached.

- ✓ **Carbonation Issues:** If bottles are not carbonating well during secondary fermentation, check seals and consider adding a small amount of sugar or fruit juice for additional fermentation activity.

Berry Bliss Kombucha offers a delicious way to enjoy the tangy sweetness of berries while reaping the health benefits of homemade probiotic-rich Kombucha. This recipe provides a simple introduction to flavoring Kombucha with fruit and can be customized with your favorite berry combinations. Enjoy the process of brewing and savoring your homemade Berry Bliss Kombucha, sharing its refreshing flavors with friends and family.

5.4 Citrus Burst Kombucha

Citrus Burst Kombucha combines the bright and tangy flavors of various citrus fruits, creating a refreshing and vitamin-packed beverage. Here's a beginner-friendly recipe to guide you through making this delightful variation of Kombucha:

Ingredients:

- ✓ **Filtered Water:** 1 gallon (about 4 liters)

- ✓ **Granulated Sugar:** 1 cup

- ✓ **Black Tea Bags:** 4-6 bags (or 2-3 tablespoons loose black tea)

- ✓ **Assorted Citrus Fruits:** 2-3 (such as oranges, lemons, limes, grapefruits)

- ✓ **Kombucha Starter Liquid:** 1-2 cups (from a previous batch or store-bought)

HOMEMADE KOMBUCHA RECIPES

✓ **SCOBY (Symbiotic Culture of Bacteria and Yeast):** 1 piece

Equipment Needed:

✓ **Large Pot:** For boiling water and steeping tea.

✓ **Glass Jar or Brewing Vessel:** 1-gallon capacity or larger, preferably glass.

✓ **Cloth Cover:** Breathable cloth (cheesecloth, paper towel, or clean cloth) secured with a rubber band.

✓ **pH Strips or pH Meter:** To monitor acidity levels during fermentation.

✓ **Bottles:** For bottling finished Kombucha (swing-top bottles are ideal).

Instructions:

1. Prepare the Sweet Tea Base:

✓ Boil 4 cups of water in a large pot.

✓ Remove from heat and stir in 1 cup of granulated sugar until dissolved.

✓ Add 4-6 black tea bags (or 2-3 tablespoons loose tea) and steep for 10-15 minutes.

- ✓ Remove the tea bags or strain loose tea and let the sweet tea mixture cool to room temperature.

2. Prepare Citrus Fruits:

- ✓ Wash and scrub the citrus fruits thoroughly under cold water to remove any dirt or wax.

- ✓ Slice the citrus fruits thinly, including the peel if desired, for a more intense citrus flavor.

3. Combine with Starter Liquid:

- ✓ Pour the cooled sweet tea into a clean glass jar or brewing vessel.

- ✓ Add the sliced citrus fruits directly into the sweet tea mixture.

4. Add Starter Liquid and SCOBY:

- ✓ Add 1-2 cups of Kombucha starter liquid from a previous batch or store-bought Kombucha.

- ✓ Gently place the SCOBY on top of the sweet tea mixture, smooth side up.

5. Fermentation:

- ✓ Cover the jar with a breathable cloth secured with a rubber band to allow airflow while keeping out insects and dust.

- ✓ Place the jar in a warm, dark place (ideally 68-85°F or 20-29°C) to ferment for 7-14 days.

- ✓ Taste-test the Kombucha after 7 days to monitor its flavor development. It should have a balanced citrusy tartness.

6. Bottling:

- ✓ Once the Kombucha reaches your desired level of tartness, carefully remove the SCOBY and set it aside in a clean container with some Kombucha starter liquid.

- ✓ Prepare your bottles by washing them thoroughly with hot water and soap, then rinsing well.

- ✓ Optionally, strain out the citrus slices and any sediment before bottling.

7. Second Fermentation (Optional):

- ✓ Pour the fermented Kombucha into bottles, leaving a few inches of headspace at the top.

✓ Seal the bottles tightly with caps or lids and place them in a warm, dark place for 1-3 days for secondary fermentation.

✓ Burp the bottles daily by gently opening them to release excess carbonation and prevent bursting.

8. Enjoy:

✓ After secondary fermentation (if performed), refrigerate the bottles to slow down carbonation and chill the Kombucha.

✓ Serve cold over ice, garnished with citrus slices if desired, and savor the refreshing citrus burst in your homemade Citrus Burst Kombucha.

Tips for Success:

✓ **Citrus Varieties:** Experiment with different combinations of citrus fruits to create unique flavor profiles.

✓ **Sanitation:** Maintain clean equipment and utensils throughout the brewing process to prevent contamination.

✓ **Temperature Control:** Ensure a stable fermentation temperature for consistent results.

Troubleshooting:

- ✓ **Fermentation Time:** If the Kombucha is too sweet after 7 days, allow it to ferment longer until it reaches the desired tartness.

- ✓ **Carbonation Issues:** If bottles are not carbonating well, check seals and consider adding a small amount of sugar or fruit juice for additional fermentation activity.

Citrus Burst Kombucha offers a refreshing and tangy variation that highlights the vibrant flavors of assorted citrus fruits. This recipe provides a simple introduction to flavoring Kombucha with citrus, allowing you to enjoy a healthful and probiotic-rich beverage at home. Experiment with different citrus combinations, adjust sweetness levels to your taste, and share the citrusy goodness of your homemade Kombucha with friends and family. Cheers to brewing and enjoying delicious Citrus Burst Kombucha!

5.5 Herbal Harmony Kombucha

Herbal Harmony Kombucha combines the soothing and aromatic notes of various herbs, offering a unique and calming twist to your homemade brew. Here's a beginner-

HOMEMADE KOMBUCHA RECIPES

friendly recipe to guide you through making this delightful variation of Kombucha:

Ingredients:

- ✓ **Filtered Water:** 1 gallon (about 4 liters)

- ✓ **Granulated Sugar:** 1 cup

- ✓ **Black Tea Bags:** 4-6 bags (or 2-3 tablespoons loose black tea)

- ✓ **Assorted Fresh Herbs:** Choose 2-3 herbs (such as mint, basil, lavender, or chamomile)

- ✓ **Kombucha Starter Liquid:** 1-2 cups (from a previous batch or store-bought)

- ✓ **SCOBY (Symbiotic Culture of Bacteria and Yeast):** 1 piece

Equipment Needed:

- ✓ **Large Pot:** For boiling water and steeping tea.

- ✓ **Glass Jar or Brewing Vessel:** 1-gallon capacity or larger, preferably glass.

- ✓ **Cloth Cover:** Breathable cloth (cheesecloth, paper towel, or clean cloth) secured with a rubber band.

- ✓ **pH Strips or pH Meter:** To monitor acidity levels during fermentation.

- ✓ **Bottles:** For bottling finished Kombucha (swing-top bottles are ideal).

Instructions:

1. Prepare the Sweet Tea Base:

- ✓ Boil 4 cups of water in a large pot.

- ✓ Remove from heat and stir in 1 cup of granulated sugar until dissolved.

- ✓ Add 4-6 black tea bags (or 2-3 tablespoons loose tea) and steep for 10-15 minutes.

- ✓ Remove the tea bags or strain loose tea and let the sweet tea mixture cool to room temperature.

2. Prepare Fresh Herbs:

- ✓ Rinse the assorted fresh herbs under cold water to remove any dirt or debris.

- ✓ If using larger herbs like basil or mint, tear or crush them gently to release their flavors.

HOMEMADE KOMBUCHA RECIPES

3. Combine with Starter Liquid:

- ✓ Pour the cooled sweet tea into a clean glass jar or brewing vessel.

- ✓ Add the assorted fresh herbs directly into the sweet tea mixture.

4. Add Starter Liquid and SCOBY:

- ✓ Add 1-2 cups of Kombucha starter liquid from a previous batch or store-bought Kombucha.

- ✓ Gently place the SCOBY on top of the sweet tea mixture, smooth side up.

5. Fermentation:

- ✓ Cover the jar with a breathable cloth secured with a rubber band to allow airflow while keeping out insects and dust.

- ✓ Place the jar in a warm, dark place (ideally 68-85°F or 20-29°C) to ferment for 7-14 days.

- ✓ Taste-test the Kombucha after 7 days to monitor its flavor development. It should have a balanced herbal infusion.

6. Bottling:

- ✓ Once the Kombucha reaches your desired level of tartness, carefully remove the SCOBY and set it aside in a clean container with some Kombucha starter liquid.

- ✓ Prepare your bottles by washing them thoroughly with hot water and soap, then rinsing well.

- ✓ Optionally, strain out the herbs and any sediment before bottling.

7. Second Fermentation (Optional):

- ✓ Pour the fermented Kombucha into bottles, leaving a few inches of headspace at the top.

- ✓ Seal the bottles tightly with caps or lids and place them in a warm, dark place for 1-3 days for secondary fermentation.

- ✓ Burp the bottles daily by gently opening them to release excess carbonation and prevent bursting.

8. Enjoy:

- ✓ After secondary fermentation (if performed), refrigerate the bottles to slow down carbonation and chill the Kombucha.

HOMEMADE KOMBUCHA RECIPES

- ✓ Serve cold over ice, garnished with fresh herbs if desired, and savor the soothing and aromatic flavors of your homemade Herbal Harmony Kombucha.

Tips for Success:

- ✓ **Herb Selection:** Experiment with different combinations of herbs to create unique flavor profiles and aromas.

- ✓ **Sanitation:** Maintain clean equipment and utensils throughout the brewing process to prevent contamination.

- ✓ **Temperature Control:** Ensure a stable fermentation temperature for consistent results.

Troubleshooting:

- ✓ **Fermentation Time:** If the Kombucha is too sweet after 7 days, allow it to ferment longer until it reaches the desired tartness.

- ✓ **Carbonation Issues:** If bottles are not carbonating well, check seals and consider adding a small amount of sugar or fruit juice for additional fermentation activity.

Herbal Harmony Kombucha offers a refreshing and aromatic variation that highlights the natural flavors and soothing properties of fresh herbs. This recipe provides a simple introduction to flavoring Kombucha with herbs, allowing you to enjoy a healthful and probiotic-rich beverage at home. Customize the herb combinations to suit your taste preferences, and share the harmonious flavors of your homemade Kombucha with friends and family. Cheers to brewing and enjoying delicious Herbal Harmony Kombucha!

CHAPTER SIX

ADVANCED RECIPES

6.1 Tropical Paradise Kombucha

Tropical Paradise Kombucha brings together the exotic flavors of tropical fruits, offering a refreshing and vibrant twist to your homemade brew. This advanced recipe involves more complex flavor combinations and techniques, perfect for Kombucha enthusiasts looking to explore unique variations. Here's a detailed guide to creating Tropical Paradise Kombucha:

Ingredients:

- ✓ **Filtered Water:** 1 gallon (about 4 liters)

- ✓ **Granulated Sugar:** 1 cup

- ✓ **Black Tea Bags:** 4-6 bags (or 2-3 tablespoons loose black tea)

- ✓ **Assorted Tropical Fruits:** Choose a mix of fruits like pineapple, mango, passion fruit, and/or kiwi (about 2 cups chopped)

- ✓ **Kombucha Starter Liquid:** 1-2 cups (from a previous batch or store-bought)

- ✓ **SCOBY (Symbiotic Culture of Bacteria and Yeast):** 1 piece

Equipment Needed:

- ✓ **Large Pot:** For boiling water and steeping tea.

- ✓ **Glass Jar or Brewing Vessel:** 1-gallon capacity or larger, preferably glass.

- ✓ **Cloth Cover:** Breathable cloth (cheesecloth, paper towel, or clean cloth) secured with a rubber band.

- ✓ **pH Strips or pH Meter:** To monitor acidity levels during fermentation.

- ✓ **Bottles:** For bottling finished Kombucha (swing-top bottles are ideal).

Instructions:

1. Prepare the Sweet Tea Base:

- ✓ Boil 4 cups of water in a large pot.

- ✓ Remove from heat and stir in 1 cup of granulated sugar until dissolved.

- ✓ Add 4-6 black tea bags (or 2-3 tablespoons loose tea) and steep for 10-15 minutes.

✓ Remove the tea bags or strain loose tea and let the sweet tea mixture cool to room temperature.

2. Prepare Tropical Fruits:

✓ Wash and peel the tropical fruits as needed.

✓ Chop the fruits into small pieces, ensuring they are ripe and flavorful.

3. Combine with Starter Liquid:

✓ Pour the cooled sweet tea into a clean glass jar or brewing vessel.

✓ Add the chopped tropical fruits directly into the sweet tea mixture.

4. Add Starter Liquid and SCOBY:

✓ Add 1-2 cups of Kombucha starter liquid from a previous batch or store-bought Kombucha.

✓ Gently place the SCOBY on top of the sweet tea mixture, smooth side up.

5. Fermentation:

✓ Cover the jar with a breathable cloth secured with a rubber band to allow airflow while keeping out insects and dust.

- ✓ Place the jar in a warm, dark place (ideally 68-85°F or 20-29°C) to ferment for 7-14 days.

- ✓ Taste-test the Kombucha after 7 days to monitor its flavor development. It should have a balanced tropical fruit infusion.

6. Bottling:

- ✓ Once the Kombucha reaches your desired level of tartness, carefully remove the SCOBY and set it aside in a clean container with some Kombucha starter liquid.

- ✓ Prepare your bottles by washing them thoroughly with hot water and soap, then rinsing well.

- ✓ Optionally, strain out the tropical fruits and any sediment before bottling.

7. Second Fermentation (Optional):

- ✓ Pour the fermented Kombucha into bottles, leaving a few inches of headspace at the top.

- ✓ Seal the bottles tightly with caps or lids and place them in a warm, dark place for 1-3 days for secondary fermentation.

HOMEMADE KOMBUCHA RECIPES

✓ Burp the bottles daily by gently opening them to release excess carbonation and prevent bursting.

8. Enjoy:

✓ After secondary fermentation (if performed), refrigerate the bottles to slow down carbonation and chill the Kombucha.

✓ Serve cold over ice, garnished with a slice of tropical fruit if desired, and savor the exotic flavors of your homemade Tropical Paradise Kombucha.

Tips for Success:

✓ **Tropical Fruit Selection:** Experiment with different combinations of tropical fruits to create unique flavor profiles.

✓ **Sanitation:** Maintain clean equipment and utensils throughout the brewing process to prevent contamination.

✓ **Temperature Control:** Ensure a stable fermentation temperature for consistent results.

Troubleshooting:

- ✓ **Fermentation Time:** If the Kombucha is too sweet after 7 days, allow it to ferment longer until it reaches the desired tartness.

- ✓ **Carbonation Issues:** If bottles are not carbonating well, check seals and consider adding a small amount of sugar or fruit juice for additional fermentation activity.

Tropical Paradise Kombucha offers an adventurous and flavorful variation that captures the essence of tropical fruits in a probiotic-rich beverage. This advanced recipe allows you to explore complex flavor combinations and refine your brewing skills. Customize the fruit combinations and fermentation techniques to suit your taste preferences, and share the tropical bliss of your homemade Kombucha with friends and family. Embrace the art of brewing and enjoy the refreshing taste of Tropical Paradise Kombucha!

6.2 Spiced Chai Kombucha

Spiced Chai Kombucha blends the rich, aromatic flavors of traditional chai spices with the tangy kick of fermented tea, creating a warm and comforting beverage. This advanced recipe introduces complex spice combinations and techniques, perfect for those seeking a flavorful twist on their homemade Kombucha. Here's a detailed guide to crafting Spiced Chai Kombucha:

Ingredients:

- ✓ **Filtered Water:** 1 gallon (about 4 liters)

- ✓ **Granulated Sugar:** 1 cup

- ✓ **Black Tea Bags:** 4-6 bags (or 2-3 tablespoons loose black tea)

- ✓ **Chai Spices:** 2-3 cinnamon sticks, 6-8 whole cloves, 6-8 cardamom pods, 1-2 inches of fresh ginger (sliced), and a pinch of black pepper

- ✓ **Kombucha Starter Liquid:** 1-2 cups (from a previous batch or store-bought)

- ✓ **SCOBY (Symbiotic Culture of Bacteria and Yeast):** 1 piece

Equipment Needed:

- ✓ **Large Pot:** For boiling water and steeping tea.

- ✓ **Glass Jar or Brewing Vessel:** 1-gallon capacity or larger, preferably glass.

- ✓ **Cloth Cover:** Breathable cloth (cheesecloth, paper towel, or clean cloth) secured with a rubber band.

- ✓ **pH Strips or pH Meter:** To monitor acidity levels during fermentation.

- ✓ **Bottles:** For bottling finished Kombucha (swing-top bottles are ideal).

Instructions:

1. Prepare the Sweet Tea Base:

- ✓ Boil 4 cups of water in a large pot.

- ✓ Remove from heat and stir in 1 cup of granulated sugar until dissolved.

- ✓ Add 4-6 black tea bags (or 2-3 tablespoons loose tea) and chai spices (cinnamon sticks, cloves, cardamom pods, sliced ginger, black pepper).

- ✓ Steep for 10-15 minutes to infuse the flavors of the chai spices into the tea.

✓ Remove the tea bags and spices or strain loose tea, allowing the sweet tea mixture to cool to room temperature.

2. Combine with Starter Liquid:

✓ Pour the cooled chai-spiced sweet tea into a clean glass jar or brewing vessel.

✓ Add 1-2 cups of Kombucha starter liquid from a previous batch or store-bought Kombucha.

3. Add SCOBY:

✓ Gently place the SCOBY on top of the sweet tea mixture, smooth side up.

4. Fermentation:

✓ Cover the jar with a breathable cloth secured with a rubber band to allow airflow while keeping out insects and dust.

✓ Place the jar in a warm, dark place (ideally 68-85°F or 20-29°C) to ferment for 7-14 days.

✓ Taste-test the Kombucha after 7 days to monitor its flavor development. It should have a balanced chai spice infusion with a hint of sweetness.

5. Bottling:

✓ Once the Kombucha reaches your desired level of tartness, carefully remove the SCOBY and set it aside in a clean container with some Kombucha starter liquid.

✓ Prepare your bottles by washing them thoroughly with hot water and soap, then rinsing well.

✓ Optionally, strain out any residual spices and sediment before bottling.

6. Second Fermentation (Optional):

✓ Pour the fermented Kombucha into bottles, leaving a few inches of headspace at the top.

✓ Seal the bottles tightly with caps or lids and place them in a warm, dark place for 1-3 days for secondary fermentation.

✓ Burp the bottles daily by gently opening them to release excess carbonation and prevent bursting.

7. Enjoy:

HOMEMADE KOMBUCHA RECIPES

- ✓ After secondary fermentation (if performed), refrigerate the bottles to slow down carbonation and chill the Kombucha.

- ✓ Serve cold over ice, garnished with a cinnamon stick or a sprinkle of ground cinnamon if desired, and savor the warming and aromatic flavors of your homemade Spiced Chai Kombucha.

Tips for Success:

- ✓ **Chai Spice Intensity:** Adjust the amount of chai spices according to your taste preferences for a stronger or milder flavor.

- ✓ **Consistency:** Maintain a stable fermentation environment and follow sanitary practices to ensure successful brewing.

- ✓ **Bottling Safety:** Use appropriate bottles and monitor carbonation levels during secondary fermentation to prevent over-carbonation.

Troubleshooting:

- ✓ **Fermentation Time:** If the Kombucha is not tart enough after 7 days, allow it to ferment longer until it reaches the desired acidity.

- ✓ **Spice Sediment:** If spices settle at the bottom of bottles, consider straining the brewed Kombucha through a fine mesh sieve before bottling.

Spiced Chai Kombucha offers a cozy and aromatic variation that combines the comforting flavors of traditional chai spices with the health benefits of homemade Kombucha. This advanced recipe invites you to experiment with complex spice combinations and enjoy the unique fusion of flavors. Share the warm and soothing essence of your homemade Spiced Chai Kombucha with friends and family, and embrace the art of brewing with this delightful beverage.

6.3 Floral Fusion Kombucha

Floral Fusion Kombucha blends the delicate and aromatic notes of edible flowers with the tangy profile of fermented tea, creating a unique and visually appealing beverage. This advanced recipe explores the infusion of floral flavors, offering a sophisticated twist on traditional Kombucha. Here's a detailed guide to crafting Floral Fusion Kombucha:

Ingredients:

HOMEMADE KOMBUCHA RECIPES

- ✓ **Filtered Water:** 1 gallon (about 4 liters)

- ✓ **Granulated Sugar:** 1 cup

- ✓ **Black Tea Bags:** 4-6 bags (or 2-3 tablespoons loose black tea)

- ✓ **Edible Flowers:** Choose a mix of edible flowers such as lavender, rose petals, hibiscus, chamomile, or jasmine (about 1 cup loosely packed)

- ✓ **Kombucha Starter Liquid:** 1-2 cups (from a previous batch or store-bought)

- ✓ **SCOBY (Symbiotic Culture of Bacteria and Yeast):** 1 piece

Equipment Needed:

- ✓ **Large Pot:** For boiling water and steeping tea.

- ✓ **Glass Jar or Brewing Vessel:** 1-gallon capacity or larger, preferably glass.

- ✓ **Cloth Cover:** Breathable cloth (cheesecloth, paper towel, or clean cloth) secured with a rubber band.

- ✓ **pH Strips or pH Meter:** To monitor acidity levels during fermentation.

HOMEMADE KOMBUCHA RECIPES

✓ **Bottles:** For bottling finished Kombucha (swing-top bottles are ideal).

Instructions:

1. Prepare the Sweet Tea Base:

✓ Boil 4 cups of water in a large pot.

✓ Remove from heat and stir in 1 cup of granulated sugar until dissolved.

✓ Add 4-6 black tea bags (or 2-3 tablespoons loose tea) and steep for 10-15 minutes.

✓ Remove the tea bags and let the sweet tea mixture cool to room temperature.

2. Prepare Edible Flowers:

✓ Rinse the edible flowers under cold water to remove any dirt or debris.

✓ Gently pat dry with a clean towel or paper towel.

3. Combine with Starter Liquid:

✓ Pour the cooled sweet tea into a clean glass jar or brewing vessel.

✓ Add the edible flowers directly into the sweet tea mixture.

HOMEMADE KOMBUCHA RECIPES

4. Add Starter Liquid and SCOBY:

- ✓ Add 1-2 cups of Kombucha starter liquid from a previous batch or store-bought Kombucha.

- ✓ Gently place the SCOBY on top of the sweet tea mixture, smooth side up.

5. Fermentation:

- ✓ Cover the jar with a breathable cloth secured with a rubber band to allow airflow while keeping out insects and dust.

- ✓ Place the jar in a warm, dark place (ideally 68-85°F or 20-29°C) to ferment for 7-14 days.

- ✓ Taste-test the Kombucha after 7 days to monitor its flavor development. It should have a delicate floral infusion with a balanced tartness.

6. Bottling:

- ✓ Once the Kombucha reaches your desired level of tartness, carefully remove the SCOBY and set it aside in a clean container with some Kombucha starter liquid.

- ✓ Prepare your bottles by washing them thoroughly with hot water and soap, then rinsing well.

✓ Optionally, strain out the edible flowers and any sediment before bottling.

7. Second Fermentation (Optional):

✓ Pour the fermented Kombucha into bottles, leaving a few inches of headspace at the top.

✓ Seal the bottles tightly with caps or lids and place them in a warm, dark place for 1-3 days for secondary fermentation.

✓ Burp the bottles daily by gently opening them to release excess carbonation and prevent bursting.

8. Enjoy:

✓ After secondary fermentation (if performed), refrigerate the bottles to slow down carbonation and chill the Kombucha.

✓ Serve cold over ice, garnished with a few fresh edible flowers if desired, and savor the delicate and aromatic flavors of your homemade Floral Fusion Kombucha.

Tips for Success:

HOMEMADE KOMBUCHA RECIPES

- ✓ **Edible Flower Selection:** Choose organic, pesticide-free edible flowers for the best flavor and safety.

- ✓ **Sanitation:** Maintain clean equipment and utensils throughout the brewing process to prevent contamination.

- ✓ **Temperature Control:** Ensure a stable fermentation temperature for consistent results.

Troubleshooting:

- ✓ **Fermentation Time:** If the Kombucha is too sweet after 7 days, allow it to ferment longer until it reaches the desired tartness.

- ✓ **Floral Aroma:** If the floral aroma is too subtle, consider adding more edible flowers or extending the steeping time during preparation.

Floral Fusion Kombucha offers a sophisticated and aromatic variation that celebrates the delicate flavors of edible flowers in a probiotic-rich beverage. This advanced recipe encourages creativity in combining floral notes with the tangy essence of Kombucha, providing a unique sensory experience. Share the floral elegance of your homemade Kombucha with friends and family, and enjoy the natural beauty and healthful benefits of Floral Fusion Kombucha.

6.4 Green Goddess Kombucha

Green Goddess Kombucha combines the fresh and vibrant flavors of green herbs and vegetables, offering a unique and healthful twist to your homemade brew. This advanced recipe focuses on using green ingredients known for their nutrient-rich profiles and refreshing taste. Here's a detailed guide to crafting Green Goddess Kombucha:

Ingredients:

- ✓ **Filtered Water:** 1 gallon (about 4 liters)

- ✓ **Granulated Sugar:** 1 cup

- ✓ **Green Tea Bags:** 4-6 bags (or 2-3 tablespoons loose green tea)

- ✓ **Fresh Green Herbs and Vegetables:** Choose a mix of green herbs (like mint, basil, cilantro) and vegetables (such as cucumber, celery) (about 2 cups chopped)

- ✓ **Kombucha Starter Liquid:** 1-2 cups (from a previous batch or store-bought)

HOMEMADE KOMBUCHA RECIPES

- ✓ **SCOBY (Symbiotic Culture of Bacteria and Yeast):** 1 piece

Equipment Needed:

- ✓ **Large Pot:** For boiling water and steeping tea.

- ✓ **Glass Jar or Brewing Vessel:** 1-gallon capacity or larger, preferably glass.

- ✓ **Cloth Cover:** Breathable cloth (cheesecloth, paper towel, or clean cloth) secured with a rubber band.

- ✓ **pH Strips or pH Meter:** To monitor acidity levels during fermentation.

- ✓ **Bottles:** For bottling finished Kombucha (swing-top bottles are ideal).

Instructions:

1. Prepare the Sweet Tea Base:

- ✓ Boil 4 cups of water in a large pot.

- ✓ Remove from heat and stir in 1 cup of granulated sugar until dissolved.

- ✓ Add 4-6 green tea bags (or 2-3 tablespoons loose green tea) and steep for 5-7 minutes.

✓ Remove the tea bags and let the sweet tea mixture cool to room temperature.

2. Prepare Fresh Green Herbs and Vegetables:

✓ Rinse the fresh green herbs and vegetables under cold water to remove any dirt or debris.

✓ Chop the herbs and vegetables into small pieces, ensuring they are fresh and vibrant.

3. Combine with Starter Liquid:

✓ Pour the cooled sweet green tea into a clean glass jar or brewing vessel.

✓ Add the chopped fresh green herbs and vegetables directly into the sweet tea mixture.

4. Add Starter Liquid and SCOBY:

✓ Add 1-2 cups of Kombucha starter liquid from a previous batch or store-bought Kombucha.

✓ Gently place the SCOBY on top of the sweet tea mixture, smooth side up.

5. Fermentation:

- ✓ Cover the jar with a breathable cloth secured with a rubber band to allow airflow while keeping out insects and dust.

- ✓ Place the jar in a warm, dark place (ideally 68-85°F or 20-29°C) to ferment for 7-14 days.

- ✓ Taste-test the Kombucha after 7 days to monitor its flavor development. It should have a fresh, green herb and vegetable infusion with a balanced tartness.

6. Bottling:

- ✓ Once the Kombucha reaches your desired level of tartness, carefully remove the SCOBY and set it aside in a clean container with some Kombucha starter liquid.

- ✓ Prepare your bottles by washing them thoroughly with hot water and soap, then rinsing well.

- ✓ Optionally, strain out the fresh green herbs, vegetables, and any sediment before bottling.

7. Second Fermentation (Optional):

✓ Pour the fermented Kombucha into bottles, leaving a few inches of headspace at the top.

✓ Seal the bottles tightly with caps or lids and place them in a warm, dark place for 1-3 days for secondary fermentation.

✓ Burp the bottles daily by gently opening them to release excess carbonation and prevent bursting.

8. Enjoy:

✓ After secondary fermentation (if performed), refrigerate the bottles to slow down carbonation and chill the Kombucha.

✓ Serve cold over ice, garnished with a fresh herb or vegetable slice if desired, and savor the invigorating and healthful flavors of your homemade Green Goddess Kombucha.

Tips for Success:

✓ **Green Ingredient Selection:** Experiment with different combinations of fresh green herbs and vegetables to create unique flavor profiles.

HOMEMADE KOMBUCHA RECIPES

✓ **Sanitation:** Maintain clean equipment and utensils throughout the brewing process to prevent contamination.

✓ **Temperature Control:** Ensure a stable fermentation temperature for consistent results.

Troubleshooting:

✓ **Fermentation Time:** If the Kombucha is too sweet after 7 days, allow it to ferment longer until it reaches the desired tartness.

✓ **Vegetable Sediment:** If vegetables settle at the bottom of bottles, consider straining the brewed Kombucha through a fine mesh sieve before bottling.

Green Goddess Kombucha offers a refreshing and nutrient-rich variation that highlights the vibrant flavors of green herbs and vegetables in a probiotic-rich beverage. This advanced recipe invites you to explore the healthful benefits and fresh taste of green ingredients, enhancing your brewing experience. Share the rejuvenating essence of your homemade Kombucha with friends and family, and enjoy the crisp and revitalizing flavors of Green Goddess Kombucha.

6.5 Decadent Dessert Kombucha

Decadent Dessert Kombucha transforms the indulgent flavors of classic desserts into a probiotic-rich beverage, offering a delightful treat with a healthy twist. This advanced recipe introduces sweet and savory elements reminiscent of popular desserts, creating a unique and satisfying drinking experience. Here's a detailed guide to crafting Decadent Dessert Kombucha:

Ingredients:

- ✓ **Filtered Water:** 1 gallon (about 4 liters)

- ✓ **Granulated Sugar:** 1 cup

- ✓ **Black Tea Bags:** 4-6 bags (or 2-3 tablespoons loose black tea)

- ✓ **Dessert Flavors:** Choose from ingredients like vanilla beans, cocoa nibs, cinnamon sticks, dried fruits (e.g., raisins, dates), or nuts (e.g., almonds, hazelnuts) (amounts vary based on preference)

- ✓ **Kombucha Starter Liquid:** 1-2 cups (from a previous batch or store-bought)

HOMEMADE KOMBUCHA RECIPES

- ✓ **SCOBY (Symbiotic Culture of Bacteria and Yeast):** 1 piece

Equipment Needed:

- ✓ **Large Pot:** For boiling water and steeping tea.

- ✓ **Glass Jar or Brewing Vessel:** 1-gallon capacity or larger, preferably glass.

- ✓ **Cloth Cover:** Breathable cloth (cheesecloth, paper towel, or clean cloth) secured with a rubber band.

- ✓ **pH Strips or pH Meter:** To monitor acidity levels during fermentation.

- ✓ **Bottles:** For bottling finished Kombucha (swing-top bottles are ideal).

Instructions:

1. Prepare the Sweet Tea Base:

- ✓ Boil 4 cups of water in a large pot.

- ✓ Remove from heat and stir in 1 cup of granulated sugar until dissolved.

- ✓ Add 4-6 black tea bags (or 2-3 tablespoons loose tea) and steep for 10-15 minutes.

✓ Remove the tea bags and let the sweet tea mixture cool to room temperature.

2. Choose Dessert Flavors:

✓ Depending on your chosen dessert theme, select and prepare ingredients such as vanilla beans (split), cocoa nibs, cinnamon sticks, dried fruits, or nuts.

✓ Consider using a combination of these ingredients to achieve the desired dessert flavor profile.

3. Combine with Starter Liquid:

✓ Pour the cooled sweet tea into a clean glass jar or brewing vessel.

✓ Add the chosen dessert flavors directly into the sweet tea mixture.

4. Add Starter Liquid and SCOBY:

✓ Add 1-2 cups of Kombucha starter liquid from a previous batch or store-bought Kombucha.

✓ Gently place the SCOBY on top of the sweet tea mixture, smooth side up.

5. Fermentation:

HOMEMADE KOMBUCHA RECIPES

✓ Cover the jar with a breathable cloth secured with a rubber band to allow airflow while keeping out insects and dust.

✓ Place the jar in a warm, dark place (ideally 68-85°F or 20-29°C) to ferment for 7-14 days.

✓ Taste-test the Kombucha after 7 days to monitor its flavor development. It should reflect the decadent dessert flavors with a balanced tartness.

6. Bottling:

✓ Once the Kombucha reaches your desired level of tartness, carefully remove the SCOBY and set it aside in a clean container with some Kombucha starter liquid.

✓ Prepare your bottles by washing them thoroughly with hot water and soap, then rinsing well.

✓ Optionally, strain out any solid ingredients and sediment before bottling.

7. Second Fermentation (Optional):

✓ Pour the fermented Kombucha into bottles, leaving a few inches of headspace at the top.

- ✓ Seal the bottles tightly with caps or lids and place them in a warm, dark place for 1-3 days for secondary fermentation.

- ✓ Burp the bottles daily by gently opening them to release excess carbonation and prevent bursting.

8. Enjoy:

- ✓ After secondary fermentation (if performed), refrigerate the bottles to slow down carbonation and chill the Kombucha.

- ✓ Serve cold over ice, garnished with a sprinkle of cocoa powder or a cinnamon stick if desired, and savor the rich and decadent flavors of your homemade Decadent Dessert Kombucha.

Tips for Success:

- ✓ **Dessert Inspiration:** Draw inspiration from your favorite desserts to create a unique flavor profile.

- ✓ **Sanitation:** Maintain clean equipment and utensils throughout the brewing process to prevent contamination.

✓ **Flavor Balance:** Adjust ingredient quantities to achieve a harmonious blend of sweet, savory, and tart flavors.

Troubleshooting:

✓ **Fermentation Time:** If the Kombucha lacks dessert flavor after 7 days, extend fermentation until the desired flavors develop.

✓ **Ingredient Sediment:** If solid ingredients settle in bottles, consider straining the brewed Kombucha through a fine mesh sieve before bottling.

Decadent Dessert Kombucha offers a creative and indulgent variation that transforms classic dessert flavors into a healthful and probiotic-rich beverage. This advanced recipe encourages experimentation with ingredients to capture the essence of your favorite desserts in a refreshing drink. Share the luscious and satisfying experience of your homemade Kombucha with friends and family, and enjoy the guilt-free pleasure of Decadent Dessert Kombucha.

CHAPTER SEVEN

KOMBUCHA FOR SENIORS

7.1 Adjusting Recipes for Senior Diets

Kombucha, a fermented tea beverage with numerous health benefits, can be tailored to suit the specific dietary needs and preferences of seniors. As individuals age, dietary requirements may change, and adjustments in recipes can ensure that Kombucha remains a safe and enjoyable addition to their wellness regimen. Here's a comprehensive look at how to adapt Kombucha recipes for seniors:

Understanding Senior Dietary Considerations

Seniors often have specific dietary considerations due to changes in metabolism, digestion, and overall health. When preparing Kombucha for seniors, it's essential to take into account the following factors:

- ✓ **Reduced Sugar Intake:** Many seniors may need to limit their sugar intake due to conditions like diabetes or to maintain overall health. Adjusting Kombucha recipes by reducing the amount of added sugar can make it suitable for seniors who are monitoring their sugar levels.

- ✓ **Low Caffeine Options:** Some seniors may be sensitive to caffeine or advised to limit their intake. Choosing teas with lower caffeine content, such as green tea or herbal teas, can be beneficial.

- ✓ **Enhancing Digestive Health:** Aging can sometimes affect digestion and nutrient absorption. Including probiotic-rich foods and beverages like Kombucha can support gut health and aid in digestion.

- ✓ **Nutrient Density:** Ensuring that Kombucha recipes are nutrient-dense can help seniors meet their dietary needs without excessive calories. Incorporating ingredients rich in vitamins, minerals, and antioxidants can contribute to overall health.

Adapting Kombucha Recipes

When modifying Kombucha recipes for seniors, consider the following adjustments:

1. Sugar Content:

- ✓ **Reduced Sugar Options:** Use less sugar during the fermentation process. While sugar is essential for feeding the SCOBY, reducing it slightly can still allow for fermentation while minimizing overall sugar content in the finished beverage.

2. Tea Selection:

✓ **Caffeine-Free or Low-Caffeine Teas:** Opt for caffeine-free herbal teas or teas with lower caffeine content, such as green tea or white tea. This helps reduce the stimulant effect while still providing beneficial compounds.

3. Flavoring Choices:

✓ **Natural Sweeteners:** If additional sweetness is desired, consider using natural sweeteners like stevia or small amounts of honey or fruit juices, which can be gentler on blood sugar levels compared to refined sugars.

4. Adding Nutrient-Rich Ingredients:

✓ **Herbs and Spices:** Incorporate herbs and spices known for their health benefits, such as ginger for digestion or turmeric for its anti-inflammatory properties.

✓ **Fruits and Vegetables:** Add fresh or dried fruits and vegetables rich in vitamins and antioxidants.

Berries, citrus fruits, and leafy greens can enhance flavor and nutritional value.

5. Monitoring Fermentation:

- ✓ **Shorter Fermentation Times:** Reduce fermentation time slightly to create a beverage that is less acidic, which may be more gentle on the stomach.

Benefits of Kombucha for Seniors

- ✓ **Digestive Support:** The probiotics in Kombucha can promote gut health and aid in digestion, which can become more challenging with age.

- ✓ **Immune Boosting:** Kombucha contains beneficial acids and antioxidants that may support immune function, helping seniors stay healthy.

- ✓ **Hydration:** As hydration needs may increase with age, Kombucha can be a flavorful way to encourage fluid intake.

Safety Considerations

- ✓ **Monitoring Sugar Levels:** Ensure that any added sugars are within dietary guidelines, especially for seniors managing conditions like diabetes.

✓ **Quality Control:** Use clean, sanitized equipment and follow safe brewing practices to prevent contamination.

✓ **Consultation:** If seniors have specific health concerns or dietary restrictions, it's advisable to consult with a healthcare provider before introducing Kombucha into their diet.

Adapting Kombucha recipes for seniors involves thoughtful consideration of their unique dietary needs and health goals. By adjusting ingredients and fermentation techniques, Kombucha can be customized to provide a flavorful and healthful beverage option that supports overall well-being in aging individuals. Experimenting with different flavors and ingredients allows seniors to enjoy the benefits of Kombucha while catering to their specific dietary preferences and health requirements.

7.2 Low Sugar Kombucha Options

For seniors and others who need to monitor their sugar intake, low sugar Kombucha options provide a balanced way to enjoy the health benefits of this fermented beverage without compromising dietary goals. Here's a detailed exploration of how to create and enjoy low sugar Kombucha:

Understanding Low Sugar Kombucha

Kombucha is traditionally made with sweetened tea that undergoes fermentation by a symbiotic culture of bacteria and yeast (SCOBY). During fermentation, the SCOBY consumes the sugars in the tea, producing organic acids, probiotics, and carbonation. However, the level of residual sugar in the finished Kombucha can vary depending on the fermentation time and ingredients used.

Tips for Making Low Sugar Kombucha

1. **Reducing Sugar in Sweet Tea:**

   ✓ Start by reducing the amount of sugar used in the initial sweet tea mixture. While sugar is necessary to feed the SCOBY during fermentation, you can use less than traditional recipes call for. Gradually decrease the amount of sugar until you find a balance that still supports fermentation but results in a less sweet final product.

2. **Choosing Low Glycemic Index Sweeteners:**

   ✓ Consider using alternative sweeteners with lower glycemic index values, such as stevia, erythritol, or monk fruit extract. These options can add sweetness without significantly impacting blood sugar levels.

3. **Shortening Fermentation Time:**

   ✓ Fermentation continues to consume sugars over time. Shortening the fermentation period can result in a Kombucha that retains more residual sweetness. Monitor the taste and acidity levels throughout the process to achieve the desired balance.

4. **Secondary Fermentation Adjustments:**

   ✓ During secondary fermentation, where flavors are infused and carbonation is enhanced, choose ingredients that add flavor without additional sugars. Fresh herbs, spices, and fruits can provide complexity without increasing sweetness.

HOMEMADE KOMBUCHA RECIPES

Recipe Ideas for Low Sugar Kombucha

- ✓ **Herbal Infusions:** Use herbs like mint, basil, or lemongrass for refreshing flavors without added sugars.

- ✓ **Citrus and Spice:** Infuse Kombucha with citrus peels (lemon, lime, orange) and spices like ginger or cinnamon for zesty, aromatic profiles.

- ✓ **Berry Blends:** Use a small amount of fresh or frozen berries (such as raspberries or blueberries) to impart fruity flavors without excessive sugars.

- ✓ **Green Tea Base:** Substitute part or all of the black tea with green tea, which typically has a lighter flavor and may require less sweetening.

Benefits of Low Sugar Kombucha

- ✓ **Blood Sugar Management:** Lower sugar content can help seniors and those with diabetes manage blood sugar levels more effectively.

- ✓ **Weight Management:** Reduced sugar intake can support weight management goals and overall health.

✓ **Digestive Health:** Probiotics in Kombucha support gut health without the need for high sugar content.

Safety Considerations

✓ **Monitoring Fermentation:** Ensure that fermentation conditions are optimal to prevent under-fermentation or contamination.

✓ **Quality Ingredients:** Use high-quality teas, sweeteners, and flavoring ingredients to maintain the integrity and health benefits of the Kombucha.

Low sugar Kombucha offers a versatile and health-conscious option for seniors and anyone seeking to reduce their sugar intake while enjoying the benefits of probiotics and natural fermentation. By experimenting with different sweeteners, fermentation times, and flavor combinations, you can create customized low sugar Kombucha recipes that suit individual tastes and dietary needs. Embrace the creativity of brewing Kombucha while prioritizing health and wellness through mindful ingredient choices and brewing techniques.

7.3 Gentle Flavors for Sensitive Palates

Seniors and individuals with sensitive palates may prefer Kombucha flavors that are mild, soothing, and easy on the taste buds. Gentle flavors can enhance the enjoyment of Kombucha while providing health benefits without overwhelming the senses. Here's a detailed exploration of gentle flavor options for sensitive palates:

Understanding Gentle Flavors in Kombucha

Gentle flavors in Kombucha are characterized by their subtle and mellow profiles, which can be achieved through careful selection of ingredients and fermentation techniques. These flavors appeal to individuals who prefer beverages that are not overly acidic, sweet, or intense in taste.

Tips for Creating Gentle Flavors

1. **Choice of Tea:**

   ✓ Opt for mild and less astringent teas such as white tea or green tea. These teas impart lighter flavors that complement delicate additions without overpowering them.

2. Minimal Sweetening:

- ✓ Use minimal amounts of sugar or alternative sweeteners to support fermentation without adding excessive sweetness. This approach allows the natural flavors of the ingredients to shine through.

3. Herbal and Floral Infusions:

- ✓ Incorporate gentle herbs and edible flowers such as chamomile, lavender, or rose petals. These ingredients add subtle floral notes that can be soothing and aromatic.

4. Citrus and Light Fruits:

- ✓ Include citrus fruits like lemon or grapefruit in moderation, as they provide refreshing acidity without dominating the overall flavor profile. Light fruits such as pear or apple can also complement gentle flavors.

5. Spices and Roots:

- ✓ Use gentle spices like cinnamon or ginger sparingly to add warmth and complexity without overwhelming the palate. Roots such as turmeric can provide earthy undertones.

Recipe Ideas for Gentle Flavors

- ✓ **Chamomile Lemon:** Brew Kombucha with chamomile tea and a touch of fresh lemon juice for a calming and citrus-infused beverage.

- ✓ **Lavender Mint:** Infuse Kombucha with dried lavender buds and fresh mint leaves to create a soothing and herbal blend.

- ✓ **Rose Petal Raspberry:** Combine Kombucha with delicate rose petals and a hint of raspberry for a floral and slightly fruity experience.

- ✓ **Ginger Pear:** Add a small amount of fresh ginger and ripe pear slices during fermentation for a gentle yet aromatic flavor profile.

Benefits of Gentle Flavors

- ✓ **Palate Sensitivity:** Gentle flavors are well-suited for individuals with sensitive palates, including seniors or those experiencing taste changes.

- ✓ **Digestive Comfort:** Mild flavors can be soothing to the digestive system, making Kombucha more enjoyable and easier to consume.

- ✓ **Aromatic Pleasure:** Herbal and floral infusions provide aromatic enjoyment, enhancing the overall drinking experience.

Safety Considerations

- ✓ **Ingredient Quality:** Ensure that all ingredients are fresh, clean, and free from contaminants to maintain the integrity of the Kombucha.

- ✓ **Fermentation Control:** Monitor fermentation times and conditions to achieve the desired flavor balance without excessive acidity.

Gentle flavors in Kombucha offer a soothing and enjoyable alternative for individuals with sensitive palates, including seniors who may appreciate milder taste profiles. By exploring gentle ingredients and infusion techniques, you can create customized Kombucha recipes that cater to specific taste preferences while providing healthful probiotic benefits. Embrace the diversity of flavors and ingredients available to craft Kombucha that is both gentle and satisfying, promoting wellness and enjoyment in every sip.

7.4 Nutrient-Boosted Recipes

Nutrient-boosted Kombucha recipes are designed to enhance the health benefits of this probiotic-rich beverage by incorporating ingredients rich in vitamins, minerals, and antioxidants. These recipes are particularly beneficial for seniors and individuals looking to maximize nutritional intake while enjoying the refreshing flavors of Kombucha. Here's a detailed exploration of nutrient-boosted Kombucha recipes:

Understanding Nutrient-Boosted Kombucha

Nutrient-boosted Kombucha focuses on using ingredients that contribute essential nutrients to support overall health and well-being. By carefully selecting nutrient-dense additions, you can elevate the nutritional profile of Kombucha while enhancing its flavor complexity.

Tips for Creating Nutrient-Boosted Recipes

1. **Incorporate Superfoods:**

✓ Add superfoods such as berries (blueberries, strawberries), leafy greens (spinach, kale), and nuts (almonds, walnuts) to enrich Kombucha with vitamins, minerals, and antioxidants.

2. Use Fresh Ingredients:

✓ Choose fresh, organic produce whenever possible to maximize nutrient content and flavor. Fresh fruits, vegetables, and herbs offer superior nutritional benefits compared to processed alternatives.

3. Variety of Colors and Textures:

✓ Aim for a diverse range of colors and textures in your ingredients. This not only enhances visual appeal but also ensures a broader spectrum of nutrients.

4. Balance Sweetness and Nutrition:

✓ Maintain a balance between sweetness and nutrition by incorporating naturally sweet fruits and vegetables while monitoring sugar content to suit dietary needs.

5. **Herbal Infusions and Spices:**

✓ Infuse Kombucha with herbs like turmeric, ginger, or cilantro, which are known for their anti-inflammatory and digestive benefits. Spices such as cinnamon or cloves can add depth and warmth.

Recipe Ideas for Nutrient-Boosted Kombucha

✓ **Berry Blast:** Combine Kombucha with a mix of antioxidant-rich berries like blueberries, raspberries, and blackberries for a vibrant and nutrient-packed beverage.

✓ **Green Goddess:** Infuse Kombucha with leafy greens such as spinach and kale, along with herbs like mint and parsley, for a detoxifying and vitamin-rich blend.

✓ **Citrus Immunity:** Add citrus fruits like oranges, lemons, and grapefruits to Kombucha, enriched with vitamin C and bioflavonoids to support immune health.

✓ **Nutty Delight:** Blend Kombucha with almonds, walnuts, or seeds (such as chia or flaxseeds) for a protein and omega-3 fatty acid boost.

Benefits of Nutrient-Boosted Kombucha

✓ **Enhanced Nutrition:** Nutrient-dense ingredients contribute vitamins, minerals, and antioxidants that support overall health, immunity, and vitality.

✓ **Bioavailability:** Combining ingredients with complementary nutrients can enhance absorption and bioavailability, maximizing the benefits of each nutrient.

✓ **Taste and Flavor Complexity:** Nutrient-boosted recipes offer diverse flavors and textures, making Kombucha enjoyable while promoting healthful benefits.

Safety Considerations

✓ **Allergies and Sensitivities:** Consider individual dietary restrictions, allergies, and sensitivities when selecting ingredients. Ensure that all ingredients are safe and suitable for consumption.

✓ **Hygiene and Cleanliness:** Maintain cleanliness throughout the brewing process to prevent contamination and ensure the safety of the final product.

Nutrient-boosted Kombucha recipes provide a flavorful and health-promoting option for seniors and individuals seeking to maximize their nutritional intake. By incorporating superfoods, fresh produce, and beneficial herbs and spices, you can create customized Kombucha blends that support overall wellness and enjoyment. Experiment with different combinations to discover nutrient-rich flavors that suit your taste preferences and dietary goals, promoting a vibrant and nourishing lifestyle through nutrient-boosted Kombucha.

7.5 Kombucha Smoothies and More

Kombucha smoothies and other creative beverages offer a delicious and nutritious way to enjoy the health benefits of Kombucha. These recipes are particularly appealing for seniors and individuals looking for refreshing, nutrient-dense options that are easy to consume and digest. Here's an in-depth exploration of how to incorporate Kombucha into smoothies and other innovative drinks:

HOMEMADE KOMBUCHA RECIPES

Understanding Kombucha Smoothies

Kombucha smoothies combine the probiotic benefits of Kombucha with the nutritional richness of fruits, vegetables, and other wholesome ingredients. These blends are not only tasty but also packed with vitamins, minerals, and antioxidants, making them a great addition to a healthy diet.

Tips for Making Kombucha Smoothies

1. **Choose Complementary Flavors:**

   - ✓ Select fruits, vegetables, and other ingredients that complement the tart and slightly sweet taste of Kombucha. Popular choices include berries, citrus fruits, leafy greens, and tropical fruits.

2. **Balance the Consistency:**

   - ✓ Adjust the consistency of your smoothie by varying the amounts of Kombucha, water, or plant-based milk. For a thicker smoothie, add yogurt, avocado, or frozen fruits.

3. **Nutrient-Dense Additions:**

✓ Enhance the nutritional value by incorporating superfoods such as chia seeds, flaxseeds, hemp seeds, or protein powders. These additions boost protein, fiber, and essential fatty acids.

4. **Natural Sweeteners:**

✓ If additional sweetness is desired, opt for natural sweeteners like honey, maple syrup, or dates. These provide a touch of sweetness without relying on refined sugars.

5. **Blending Techniques:**

✓ Blend ingredients gradually, starting with the liquid base (Kombucha) and adding solids progressively. This ensures a smooth, well-mixed beverage.

Recipe Ideas for Kombucha Smoothies

✓ **Berry Kombucha Smoothie:**

➢ Ingredients: 1 cup Kombucha, 1 cup mixed berries (strawberries, blueberries, raspberries), 1 banana, 1 tablespoon chia seeds, 1/2 cup Greek yogurt.

HOMEMADE KOMBUCHA RECIPES

> Instructions: Blend all ingredients until smooth. Serve immediately.

✓ **Tropical Green Kombucha Smoothie:**

> Ingredients: 1 cup Kombucha, 1/2 cup pineapple chunks, 1/2 cup mango chunks, 1 cup spinach, 1/2 avocado, juice of 1 lime.

> Instructions: Blend all ingredients until smooth. Adjust sweetness with a touch of honey if desired.

✓ **Citrus Ginger Kombucha Smoothie:**

> Ingredients: 1 cup Kombucha, 1 orange (peeled and segmented), 1/2 cup carrots (chopped), 1 small piece of fresh ginger, 1/2 cup coconut water.

> Instructions: Blend all ingredients until smooth. Add ice cubes for a chilled effect.

✓ **Nutty Banana Kombucha Smoothie:**

> Ingredients: 1 cup Kombucha, 1 banana, 2 tablespoons almond butter, 1/2 cup almond milk, 1 tablespoon flaxseeds.

HOMEMADE KOMBUCHA RECIPES

> ➢ Instructions: Blend all ingredients until smooth. Garnish with a sprinkle of cinnamon.

Beyond Smoothies: Creative Kombucha Beverages

- ✓ **Kombucha Mocktails:**

  > ➢ Mix Kombucha with sparkling water, fresh fruit juices, and herbs like mint or basil for refreshing non-alcoholic cocktails.

- ✓ **Kombucha Iced Teas:**

  > ➢ Combine Kombucha with brewed herbal or green teas, sweetened with a touch of honey or agave syrup. Serve over ice with lemon slices.

- ✓ **Kombucha Slushies:**

  > ➢ Blend Kombucha with ice and your choice of fruits for a cool and refreshing slushy. Perfect for hot days.

- ✓ **Kombucha Popsicles:**

HOMEMADE KOMBUCHA RECIPES

> ➤ Pour Kombucha mixed with fruit puree into popsicle molds and freeze. These make for a healthy and refreshing treat.

Benefits of Kombucha Smoothies and Beverages

✓ **Digestive Health:** The probiotics in Kombucha support gut health and digestion, which can be beneficial for seniors and individuals with digestive concerns.

✓ **Nutrient-Rich:** Smoothies and other beverages can be tailored to include a wide range of nutrients, supporting overall health and wellness.

✓ **Hydration:** These beverages contribute to daily hydration needs, which is especially important for seniors who may need to increase fluid intake.

Safety Considerations

✓ **Quality Ingredients:** Ensure all ingredients, especially Kombucha, are fresh and high-quality. Avoid using Kombucha that has been improperly stored or fermented for too long.

✓ **Allergies and Sensitivities:** Be mindful of potential allergies and sensitivities when selecting ingredients. Customize recipes to accommodate individual dietary restrictions.

Kombucha smoothies and other creative beverages offer a versatile and enjoyable way to incorporate the health benefits of Kombucha into a daily diet. By experimenting with different ingredients and flavor combinations, you can create refreshing and nutrient-dense drinks that cater to various taste preferences and dietary needs. Embrace the creativity and health benefits of Kombucha beverages, making them a delightful part of your wellness routine.

CHAPTER EIGHT

KOMBUCHA AND HEALTH

8.1 Kombucha for Digestion

Kombucha, a fermented tea beverage, has gained significant attention for its potential health benefits, particularly in supporting digestive health. This chapter delves into the digestive benefits of Kombucha, exploring the scientific basis, potential mechanisms, and practical applications for improving digestive wellness.

The Digestive Benefits of Kombucha

1. Probiotic Content:

- ✓ **Role of Probiotics:** Kombucha is rich in probiotics, which are beneficial bacteria that contribute to gut health. Probiotics help maintain a healthy balance of gut microbiota, which is crucial for optimal digestion and overall health.

- ✓ **Common Probiotics in Kombucha:** Kombucha typically contains strains of bacteria such as Lactobacillus and Bifidobacterium, which are known for their positive effects on gut health.

HOMEMADE KOMBUCHA RECIPES

2. Organic Acids:

- ✓ **Acetic Acid:** Produced during fermentation, acetic acid helps regulate stomach acidity and can inhibit the growth of harmful bacteria, promoting a healthier gut environment.

- ✓ **Lactic Acid:** Another byproduct of fermentation, lactic acid aids in the digestion of lactose and supports the growth of beneficial gut bacteria.

3. Digestive Enzymes:

- ✓ **Enzyme Production:** The fermentation process in Kombucha produces enzymes that assist in breaking down food, making nutrients more accessible and improving overall digestion.

- ✓ **Specific Enzymes:** Kombucha can contain enzymes such as amylase, protease, and lipase, which help in the digestion of carbohydrates, proteins, and fats, respectively.

4. Antioxidants and Polyphenols:

- ✓ **Source of Antioxidants:** The tea used in Kombucha, especially green tea, is rich in polyphenols and antioxidants. These compounds help reduce oxidative stress and inflammation in the gut, which can improve digestive health.

✓ **Polyphenol Benefits:** Polyphenols promote the growth of beneficial gut bacteria and inhibit harmful pathogens, supporting a balanced gut microbiome.

How Kombucha Supports Digestive Health

1. Enhancing Gut Flora:

✓ **Microbiome Balance:** The probiotics in Kombucha help restore and maintain a healthy balance of gut flora. This balance is essential for efficient digestion, nutrient absorption, and immune function.

✓ **Prebiotic Effects:** Some components of Kombucha may act as prebiotics, providing nourishment for beneficial bacteria in the gut and enhancing their activity.

2. Improving Bowel Regularity:

✓ **Constipation Relief:** Regular consumption of Kombucha can help alleviate constipation by promoting bowel regularity. The probiotics and organic acids stimulate peristalsis, the muscle contractions that move food through the digestive tract.

✓ **Digestive Ease:** For individuals with irritable bowel syndrome (IBS) or other digestive disorders, Kombucha may help ease symptoms such as bloating, gas, and irregular bowel movements.

3. Supporting Immune Function:

✓ **Gut-Immune Connection:** A significant portion of the immune system resides in the gut. By promoting a healthy gut microbiome, Kombucha can indirectly support immune function, helping the body fend off infections and illnesses.

✓ **Anti-Inflammatory Properties:** The antioxidants and polyphenols in Kombucha have anti-inflammatory effects, which can reduce gut inflammation and improve overall digestive health.

4. Detoxification:

✓ **Liver Support:** Kombucha contains glucuronic acid, which is believed to support liver detoxification. The liver plays a crucial role in filtering toxins from the blood, and a healthy liver contributes to better digestion.

✓ **Toxin Binding:** The enzymes and acids in Kombucha may help bind and eliminate toxins from the digestive tract, promoting a cleaner and more efficient digestive system.

Practical Tips for Using Kombucha to Support Digestion

1. Starting Slowly:

✓ **Gradual Introduction:** For those new to Kombucha, it's essential to start with small amounts and gradually increase intake. This allows the body to adjust to the influx of probiotics and prevents digestive discomfort.

✓ **Recommended Amount:** Begin with about 4-6 ounces per day and slowly increase to 8-12 ounces, depending on individual tolerance and digestive response.

2. Consistency and Moderation:

✓ **Regular Consumption:** Consistent, moderate consumption of Kombucha is key to reaping its digestive benefits. Incorporate it into your daily routine to support ongoing gut health.

✓ **Avoiding Excess:** While Kombucha is beneficial, excessive consumption can lead to digestive upset or excess calorie intake. Balance is crucial for optimal benefits.

3. Pairing with Meals:

✓ **Enhancing Digestion:** Drinking Kombucha with meals can aid in digestion by providing digestive enzymes and probiotics that assist in breaking down food.

✓ **Timing Considerations:** Some individuals may prefer consuming Kombucha before meals to stimulate appetite and digestive juices, while others may find it more beneficial after meals to aid in digestion.

4. Listening to Your Body:

✓ **Personal Tolerance:** Pay attention to how your body responds to Kombucha. While many people experience improved digestion, some may find it too acidic or experience mild digestive discomfort initially.

- ✓ **Adjusting Intake:** Adjust the amount and frequency of Kombucha consumption based on your digestive comfort and overall health goals.

Kombucha offers a natural and effective way to support digestive health through its rich content of probiotics, organic acids, enzymes, and antioxidants. By enhancing gut flora, improving bowel regularity, supporting immune function, and aiding in detoxification, Kombucha can be a valuable addition to a digestive wellness regimen. Embrace the benefits of Kombucha by incorporating it into your diet mindfully, listening to your body, and enjoying the journey to better digestive health.

8.2 Boosting Immunity with Kombucha

Kombucha, known for its probiotic-rich composition and various health-promoting properties, has been suggested to have immune-boosting benefits. This section explores how Kombucha can support and enhance the immune system, focusing on its components and their mechanisms of action.

Understanding Immunity and Kombucha

The immune system is the body's defense against infections and illnesses, involving various cells, tissues, and organs that work together to identify and neutralize harmful invaders like bacteria, viruses, and toxins. A healthy immune system is essential for maintaining overall health and well-being. Kombucha, through its unique blend of probiotics, antioxidants, and other bioactive compounds, can play a role in supporting immune function.

Key Components of Kombucha for Immune Health

1. Probiotics:

- ✓ **Gut-Immune Connection:** The gut microbiome plays a crucial role in the immune system. Probiotics in Kombucha, such as Lactobacillus and Bifidobacterium, help maintain a healthy gut microbiota, which is vital for a robust immune response.

- ✓ **Enhancing Immune Cells:** Probiotics can influence the activity of immune cells, such as macrophages, natural killer cells, and T lymphocytes, enhancing their ability to fight infections.

2. Antioxidants:

- ✓ **Free Radical Scavenging:** Kombucha, especially when made with green or black tea, contains antioxidants like polyphenols and catechins. These compounds neutralize free radicals, reducing oxidative stress and inflammation, which can otherwise weaken the immune system.

✓ **Supporting Immune Cells:** Antioxidants protect immune cells from damage, ensuring they function optimally.

3. Organic Acids:

✓ **Acetic Acid and Immunity:** Acetic acid, a major component of Kombucha, has antimicrobial properties that can help protect the body against harmful pathogens.

✓ **Lactic Acid and Gut Health:** Lactic acid aids in maintaining an acidic environment in the gut, which discourages the growth of harmful bacteria and supports beneficial ones.

4. Vitamins and Minerals:

✓ **Vitamin C:** Some Kombucha recipes include fruits rich in vitamin C, a vital nutrient for immune health. Vitamin C enhances the production and function of white blood cells, the body's primary defense against infections.

- ✓ **B Vitamins:** Kombucha contains B vitamins, which support energy metabolism and the production of immune cells.

Mechanisms of Immune Support

1. Modulating the Gut Microbiome:

- ✓ **Microbiome Balance:** The probiotics in Kombucha help maintain a healthy balance of gut bacteria, which is essential for immune regulation. A balanced gut microbiome enhances the body's ability to distinguish between harmful pathogens and beneficial microbes.

- ✓ **Barrier Function:** A healthy gut microbiome supports the integrity of the gut barrier, preventing the translocation of harmful pathogens into the bloodstream.

2. Reducing Inflammation:

- ✓ **Anti-Inflammatory Effects:** Chronic inflammation can weaken the immune system. The antioxidants and polyphenols in Kombucha help reduce inflammation, supporting overall immune health.

✓ **Inflammatory Mediators:** Probiotics can modulate the production of cytokines, signaling molecules that regulate inflammation and immune responses.

3. Enhancing Immune Cell Function:

✓ **Activation and Proliferation:** Probiotics in Kombucha can enhance the activation and proliferation of various immune cells, including macrophages, natural killer cells, and T lymphocytes.

✓ **Antimicrobial Activity:** Organic acids and other bioactive compounds in Kombucha exhibit antimicrobial activity, helping the immune system fight off infections more effectively.

Practical Tips for Using Kombucha to Boost Immunity

1. Consistent Consumption:

✓ **Daily Intake:** Regular consumption of Kombucha can help maintain a steady supply of beneficial probiotics, antioxidants, and other immune-supporting compounds.

✓ **Moderate Amounts:** Consuming 4-8 ounces of Kombucha daily is generally sufficient to support immune health without overwhelming the digestive system.

2. Choosing the Right Ingredients:

- ✓ **High-Quality Tea:** Use high-quality green or black tea to maximize the antioxidant content.

- ✓ **Immune-Boosting Additions:** Consider adding ingredients like ginger, turmeric, and citrus fruits, which are known for their immune-boosting properties.

3. Monitoring Sugar Content:

- ✓ **Balanced Sweetness:** Ensure that the Kombucha is not overly sweet, as high sugar intake can negatively affect immune function. Proper fermentation reduces sugar content while retaining beneficial properties.

4. Listening to Your Body:

- ✓ **Individual Responses:** Pay attention to how your body responds to Kombucha. Some individuals may experience digestive adjustments initially, which can normalize with consistent use.

✓ **Allergy Considerations:** Be mindful of any allergies or sensitivities to ingredients used in Kombucha.

Kombucha can be a valuable addition to a diet aimed at boosting immunity. Its rich content of probiotics, antioxidants, organic acids, and vitamins contributes to a healthy gut microbiome, reduces inflammation, and enhances immune cell function. By incorporating Kombucha into your daily routine, you can support your immune system naturally, promoting better overall health and resilience against infections. Remember to consume Kombucha mindfully and enjoy its refreshing taste while reaping its immune-boosting benefits.

8.3 Kombucha and Detoxification

Kombucha is often touted for its detoxifying properties, attributed to its unique composition of probiotics, organic acids, enzymes, and antioxidants. Detoxification is the body's natural process of removing toxins and waste products. This section explores how Kombucha can support and enhance the body's detoxification processes.

HOMEMADE KOMBUCHA RECIPES

The Detoxification Process

Detoxification involves several organs and systems, primarily the liver, kidneys, intestines, lungs, and skin. The liver is the central organ in detoxification, breaking down toxins into less harmful substances that can be excreted. Supporting these organs and systems can enhance the body's ability to detoxify efficiently.

Key Components of Kombucha for Detoxification

1. Probiotics:

- ✓ **Gut Health:** Probiotics in Kombucha help maintain a healthy gut microbiome, which plays a crucial role in detoxification. A balanced gut microbiome aids in the elimination of toxins through regular bowel movements and prevents the reabsorption of toxins.

- ✓ **Reduction of Pathogens:** Probiotics can outcompete harmful bacteria and yeast, reducing the production of toxic byproducts in the gut.

2. Organic Acids:

- ✓ **Acetic Acid:** This organic acid helps maintain an acidic environment in the gut, which inhibits the growth of pathogenic bacteria and promotes the growth of beneficial bacteria.

✓ **Glucuronic Acid:** Kombucha contains glucuronic acid, a compound that binds to toxins in the liver, transforming them into water-soluble forms that can be excreted through urine.

✓ **Lactic Acid:** Lactic acid aids in the detoxification process by supporting the growth of lactobacilli in the gut, which can help break down and remove waste products.

3. Antioxidants:

✓ **Free Radical Neutralization:** Kombucha, especially when made with green or black tea, is rich in antioxidants like polyphenols and catechins. These antioxidants neutralize free radicals, reducing oxidative stress that can damage cells and impair detoxification.

✓ **Support for Detox Enzymes:** Antioxidants support the activity of detoxification enzymes in the liver, enhancing the body's ability to process and eliminate toxins.

HOMEMADE KOMBUCHA RECIPES

4. Enzymes:

- ✓ **Digestive Enzymes:** The fermentation process in Kombucha produces enzymes that aid in digestion, helping to break down food and reduce the burden on the digestive system.

- ✓ **Detoxification Enzymes:** Enzymes such as glucuronyl transferase, produced during Kombucha fermentation, support the liver's detoxification pathways.

5. Polyphenols and Catechins:

- ✓ **Protective Effects:** These compounds help protect the liver from damage and enhance its detoxification capacity.

- ✓ **Anti-inflammatory Properties:** Polyphenols and catechins reduce inflammation, which can support the detoxification process by reducing the burden on detox organs.

How Kombucha Supports Detoxification

1. Liver Detoxification:

- ✓ **Phase I and Phase II Detoxification:** The liver detoxifies toxins through two phases. Kombucha supports both phases by providing glucuronic acid for conjugation (Phase II) and antioxidants that reduce oxidative stress (Phase I).

✓ **Enhanced Excretion:** Glucuronic acid in Kombucha helps in converting fat-soluble toxins into water-soluble forms, facilitating their excretion through urine and bile.

2. Digestive Health:

✓ **Regular Bowel Movements:** Probiotics and organic acids in Kombucha promote regular bowel movements, which are essential for the elimination of waste and toxins from the body.

✓ **Gut Barrier Integrity:** A healthy gut microbiome supported by Kombucha strengthens the gut barrier, preventing the reabsorption of toxins and harmful substances.

3. Immune System Support:

✓ **Modulating Inflammation:** By reducing inflammation, Kombucha helps maintain a healthy immune system, which is crucial for identifying and eliminating harmful substances.

✓ **Detox Pathways:** The immune system plays a role in detoxification by identifying and removing foreign substances. Kombucha supports immune function through its probiotic and antioxidant content.

4. Hydration:

✓ **Hydration Aid:** Kombucha contributes to daily hydration, which is essential for the kidneys to filter and excrete toxins effectively.

✓ **Diuretic Properties:** The slight diuretic effect of Kombucha can help in flushing out toxins through increased urine production.

Practical Tips for Using Kombucha for Detoxification

1. Regular Consumption:

✓ **Consistent Intake:** Incorporate Kombucha into your daily routine to support ongoing detoxification processes. Aim for 4-8 ounces per day, adjusting based on your body's response.

✓ **Balanced Diet:** Combine Kombucha consumption with a balanced diet rich in fruits, vegetables, and whole grains to enhance detoxification.

HOMEMADE KOMBUCHA RECIPES

2. Choosing the Right Kombucha:

- ✓ **Quality Ingredients:** Use high-quality tea and pure water to brew Kombucha. Organic ingredients reduce the risk of introducing additional toxins.

- ✓ **Flavor Additions:** Enhance detoxification benefits by adding ingredients like ginger, lemon, and turmeric, which are known for their detoxifying properties.

3. Mindful Brewing:

- ✓ **Proper Fermentation:** Ensure proper fermentation to maximize the production of beneficial compounds while minimizing potential contaminants.

- ✓ **Hygiene and Cleanliness:** Maintain cleanliness throughout the brewing process to avoid contamination and ensure the safety of the final product.

4. Listening to Your Body:

- ✓ **Individual Tolerance:** Monitor how your body responds to Kombucha. If you experience any adverse effects, adjust the amount or frequency of consumption.

✓ **Gradual Introduction:** Start with small amounts if you're new to Kombucha to allow your body to adjust to the influx of probiotics and organic acids.

Kombucha can be a valuable ally in supporting the body's natural detoxification processes. Its rich content of probiotics, organic acids, antioxidants, and enzymes contributes to liver detoxification, digestive health, and overall immune function. By incorporating Kombucha into your daily routine mindfully, you can enhance your body's ability to detoxify and maintain optimal health. Remember to consume Kombucha in moderation, choose high-quality ingredients, and listen to your body's signals to maximize its detoxifying benefits.

8.4 Understanding Probiotics

Probiotics are live microorganisms that confer health benefits to the host when consumed in adequate amounts. They are commonly found in fermented foods like yogurt, sauerkraut, kimchi, and kombucha. This section explores the role of probiotics in health, focusing on their mechanisms of action, benefits, and how Kombucha serves as a source of these beneficial microbes.

What Are Probiotics?

Probiotics are often referred to as "good" or "friendly" bacteria because they help maintain the balance of microorganisms in the gut, contributing to overall health. The most commonly studied probiotic strains belong to the Lactobacillus and Bifidobacterium genera, although many other types exist.

Key Probiotic Strains

1. **Lactobacillus:**

   ✓ **Functions:** Lactobacillus species produce lactic acid, which helps create an acidic environment in the gut, inhibiting the growth of harmful bacteria. They also aid in the digestion of lactose, improving tolerance to dairy products.

   ✓ **Health Benefits:** Lactobacillus probiotics can enhance gut health, boost the immune system, and may help in managing conditions like irritable bowel syndrome (IBS) and diarrhea.

2. **Bifidobacterium:**

   ✓ **Functions:** Bifidobacterium species are prominent in the intestines, especially in infants. They play a crucial role in breaking down dietary fiber, producing short-chain fatty acids that nourish the gut lining.

   ✓ **Health Benefits:** These probiotics are known for improving digestion, reducing inflammation, and supporting immune function.

3. **Saccharomyces boulardii:**

   ✓ **Functions:** This yeast probiotic helps combat pathogens in the gut and supports intestinal health.

   ✓ **Health Benefits:** It is effective in preventing and treating antibiotic-associated diarrhea and may help with certain gastrointestinal conditions.

How Probiotics Work

1. Balancing the Gut Microbiota:

- ✓ **Competitive Exclusion:** Probiotics compete with pathogenic bacteria for nutrients and adhesion sites on the gut lining, preventing harmful bacteria from establishing.

- ✓ **Antimicrobial Production:** Probiotics produce substances like lactic acid, hydrogen peroxide, and bacteriocins that inhibit the growth of pathogens.

2. Enhancing Gut Barrier Function:

- ✓ **Tight Junctions:** Probiotics strengthen the gut barrier by enhancing the integrity of tight junctions between epithelial cells, preventing the leakage of harmful substances into the bloodstream.

- ✓ **Mucus Production:** They stimulate the production of mucus, which acts as a protective layer in the gut.

3. Modulating the Immune System:

✓ **Immune Activation:** Probiotics interact with gut-associated lymphoid tissue (GALT) to modulate immune responses. They can enhance the activity of immune cells like macrophages, dendritic cells, and T lymphocytes.

✓ **Anti-Inflammatory Effects:** Probiotics can reduce inflammation by modulating the production of cytokines, signaling molecules that regulate immune responses.

4. Metabolite Production:

✓ **Short-Chain Fatty Acids (SCFAs):** Probiotics ferment dietary fibers to produce SCFAs like butyrate, propionate, and acetate. These SCFAs provide energy to colon cells, reduce inflammation, and improve gut health.

✓ **Vitamin Synthesis:** Certain probiotics synthesize vitamins like B12 and K, contributing to nutritional health.

Health Benefits of Probiotics

1. Digestive Health:

✓ **Diarrhea Prevention and Treatment:** Probiotics are effective in preventing and treating various types of diarrhea, including antibiotic-associated and traveler's diarrhea.

✓ **Irritable Bowel Syndrome (IBS):** Probiotics can help alleviate symptoms of IBS, such as bloating, gas, and abdominal pain.

2. Immune Support:

✓ **Infection Prevention:** Probiotics can reduce the risk of respiratory and gastrointestinal infections by enhancing the immune response.

✓ **Allergy Reduction:** They may help reduce the incidence and severity of allergies by modulating the immune system.

3. Mental Health:

✓ **Gut-Brain Axis:** Probiotics influence the gut-brain axis, potentially improving mental health conditions like depression and anxiety through the production of neurotransmitters and anti-inflammatory molecules.

4. Metabolic Health:

✓ **Weight Management:** Probiotics may support weight management by influencing the gut microbiota composition and metabolic processes.

✓ **Blood Sugar Control:** They can improve blood sugar levels and insulin sensitivity, contributing to better metabolic health.

Kombucha as a Source of Probiotics

1. Fermentation Process:

✓ **Symbiotic Culture of Bacteria and Yeast (SCOBY):** Kombucha is made by fermenting sweetened tea with a SCOBY, a combination of bacteria and yeast. This fermentation process produces various probiotic strains.

✓ **Microbial Diversity:** Kombucha contains a diverse array of probiotics, including species from Lactobacillus, Gluconobacter, and Zygosaccharomyces.

2. Health Benefits:

✓ **Gut Health:** Regular consumption of Kombucha can support gut health by introducing beneficial probiotics that help balance the gut microbiota.

- ✓ **Immune Support:** The probiotics in Kombucha can enhance the immune system, helping the body to fight off infections and illnesses.

- ✓ **Detoxification:** Probiotics in Kombucha aid in detoxification by promoting regular bowel movements and supporting liver function.

3. Considerations:

- ✓ **Fermentation Time:** The length of fermentation affects the probiotic content of Kombucha. Longer fermentation periods can increase the concentration of beneficial microbes.

- ✓ **Storage and Handling:** Proper storage and handling of Kombucha are essential to preserve its probiotic content. Refrigeration helps maintain the viability of probiotics.

Practical Tips for Maximizing Probiotic Benefits from Kombucha

1. Regular Consumption:

- ✓ **Daily Intake:** Incorporate Kombucha into your daily routine to ensure a consistent supply of probiotics. Start with small amounts (4-8 ounces) and gradually increase based on tolerance.

- ✓ **Diverse Diet:** Combine Kombucha with other probiotic-rich foods like yogurt, kefir, and sauerkraut to diversify your probiotic intake.

2. Proper Brewing Techniques:

- ✓ **Quality Ingredients:** Use high-quality tea and sugar to brew Kombucha, ensuring a healthy fermentation process.

- ✓ **Clean Environment:** Maintain a clean brewing environment to prevent contamination and ensure the safety of the final product.

3. Flavor Additions:

- ✓ **Nutrient Boost:** Enhance Kombucha with fruits, herbs, and spices known for their health benefits, like ginger, turmeric, and berries.

- ✓ **Custom Blends:** Experiment with different flavor combinations to create a delicious and health-promoting beverage.

Probiotics are essential for maintaining gut health, supporting the immune system, and contributing to overall well-being. Kombucha, as a rich source of diverse probiotics, offers a natural and enjoyable way to boost your intake of these beneficial microbes. By understanding the mechanisms of probiotics and incorporating Kombucha into your diet, you can enhance your digestive health, strengthen your immune system, and support your body's natural detoxification processes. Remember to consume Kombucha mindfully, practice proper brewing techniques, and enjoy the journey to better health through probiotics.

CHAPTER NINE

KOMBUCHA BEYOND THE GLASS

9.1 Cooking with Kombucha

Kombucha, a fermented tea drink packed with probiotics, enzymes, and antioxidants, has gained popularity not only as a beverage but also as a versatile ingredient in cooking. Its unique flavor profile, ranging from tangy and slightly sweet to intensely sour, makes it a creative addition to a variety of dishes. In this chapter, we will explore the innovative ways to incorporate Kombucha into your cooking, enhancing both flavor and nutritional value.

The Versatility of Kombucha in Cooking

Kombucha's complexity in flavor and acidity makes it an excellent substitute for vinegar, citrus, or even wine in recipes. Its use can span across different types of dishes, from savory to sweet, and can be employed in various culinary techniques such as marinating, glazing, baking, and fermenting.

Benefits of Cooking with Kombucha

1. **Enhanced Flavor Profiles:**

    ✓ **Tanginess and Depth:** Kombucha's natural acidity and slight effervescence can add a depth of flavor to dishes, balancing sweetness and richness.

    ✓ **Complexity:** The fermentation process gives Kombucha a unique taste, often described as a combination of cider and tea, which can elevate the overall flavor profile of your meals.

2. **Nutritional Boost:**

    ✓ **Probiotics:** While cooking might reduce the number of live probiotics, some beneficial bacteria can survive, and their metabolic by-products can still offer health benefits.

    ✓ **Antioxidants:** Kombucha retains its antioxidants even when heated, contributing to the nutritional value of your dishes.

3. **Natural Tenderizer:**

- ✓ **Enzymatic Action:** The enzymes present in Kombucha can help break down proteins in meat, making it an effective tenderizer for marinating.

Culinary Applications of Kombucha

1. Marinades:

- ✓ **Meat and Poultry:** Kombucha can be used as a base for marinades, imparting flavor while tenderizing the meat. Combine Kombucha with herbs, spices, and a bit of oil for a balanced marinade.

- ✓ **Vegetables:** Use Kombucha to marinate vegetables before grilling or roasting to add a tangy twist and enhance their natural flavors.

2. Salad Dressings:

- ✓ **Vinaigrettes:** Replace vinegar with Kombucha in your vinaigrette recipes for a milder, more complex flavor. Mix with olive oil, mustard, honey, and herbs for a refreshing salad dressing.

✓ **Creamy Dressings:** Blend Kombucha with yogurt, garlic, and dill to create a probiotic-rich, creamy dressing for salads and bowls.

3. Sauces and Glazes:

✓ **Barbecue Sauce:** Add Kombucha to your barbecue sauce for a tangy kick. Its acidity can help balance the sweetness of the sauce, adding depth and complexity.

✓ **Glazes:** Use Kombucha as a base for glazes, combining it with ingredients like honey, soy sauce, and ginger for a flavorful coating on meats or vegetables.

4. Baking:

✓ **Bread and Dough:** Incorporate Kombucha into bread or dough recipes as a substitute for part of the liquid. Its acidity can enhance the dough's fermentation, resulting in a tangy and slightly airy texture.

✓ **Cakes and Muffins:** Use Kombucha in cake or muffin batters to add moisture and a subtle tanginess. It pairs well with fruity and citrus flavors.

5. Fermented Foods:

✓ **Pickles:** Kombucha can be used as a brine for pickling vegetables. Its acidity creates an ideal environment for fermentation, resulting in tangy, probiotic-rich pickles.

✓ **Sourdough Starter:** Incorporate Kombucha into your sourdough starter for an extra boost of fermentation activity and unique flavor.

6. Beverages:

✓ **Mocktails:** Combine Kombucha with fruit juices, sparkling water, and fresh herbs to create refreshing, non-alcoholic mocktails.

✓ **Cocktails:** Use Kombucha as a mixer in cocktails, adding a probiotic twist and complexity to traditional drinks.

Recipes Featuring Kombucha

1. Kombucha-Marinated Chicken:

✓ **Ingredients:**

➢ 1 cup Kombucha

➢ 2 tablespoons olive oil

- ➢ 2 cloves garlic, minced

- ➢ 1 tablespoon honey

- ➢ 1 teaspoon dried thyme

- ➢ Salt and pepper to taste

- ➢ 4 chicken breasts

✓ **Instructions:**

1. In a bowl, combine Kombucha, olive oil, garlic, honey, thyme, salt, and pepper.

2. Place the chicken breasts in a resealable bag and pour the marinade over them.

3. Seal the bag and refrigerate for at least 4 hours or overnight.

4. Preheat the grill to medium-high heat and cook the chicken until it reaches an internal temperature of 165°F (75°C), about 6-7 minutes per side.

2. Kombucha Vinaigrette:

✓ **Ingredients:**

- ➢ 1/2 cup Kombucha

- ➢ 1/4 cup olive oil

HOMEMADE KOMBUCHA RECIPES

- ➢ 1 tablespoon Dijon mustard

- ➢ 1 tablespoon honey

- ➢ Salt and pepper to taste

- ➢ 1 tablespoon chopped fresh herbs (e.g., parsley, basil)

✓ **Instructions:**

1. In a jar with a tight-fitting lid, combine Kombucha, olive oil, Dijon mustard, honey, salt, pepper, and herbs.

2. Shake well until the ingredients are fully emulsified.

3. Drizzle over mixed greens or roasted vegetables.

3. Kombucha-BBQ Glazed Ribs:

✓ **Ingredients:**

- ➢ 1 cup Kombucha

- ➢ 1/2 cup ketchup

- ➢ 1/4 cup brown sugar

- ➢ 2 tablespoons soy sauce

- ➢ 2 tablespoons apple cider vinegar

- ➢ 1 teaspoon smoked paprika

> ➢ 1 teaspoon garlic powder

> ➢ 1 rack of baby back ribs

✓ **Instructions:**

1. Preheat the oven to 300°F (150°C).

2. In a saucepan, combine Kombucha, ketchup, brown sugar, soy sauce, vinegar, smoked paprika, and garlic powder. Simmer until thickened, about 15 minutes.

3. Place the ribs on a baking sheet, brush with the Kombucha-BBQ sauce, and cover with foil.

4. Bake for 2.5 to 3 hours, basting with more sauce every 30 minutes.

5. Finish on the grill or under the broiler for a few minutes to caramelize the glaze.

4. Kombucha Sourdough Bread:

✓ **Ingredients:**

> ➢ 1 cup Kombucha

> ➢ 1 cup sourdough starter

> ➢ 3 cups bread flour

> ➢ 1 teaspoon salt

HOMEMADE KOMBUCHA RECIPES

> ➢ 1/2 cup water (as needed)

✓ **Instructions:**

1. In a large bowl, combine Kombucha, sourdough starter, bread flour, and salt.

2. Mix until a shaggy dough forms, adding water as needed to achieve the right consistency.

3. Knead the dough on a floured surface until smooth and elastic.

4. Place the dough in a greased bowl, cover, and let rise until doubled in size, about 4-6 hours.

5. Preheat the oven to 450°F (230°C) with a Dutch oven inside.

6. Shape the dough into a round loaf, place it in the hot Dutch oven, cover, and bake for 30 minutes.

7. Remove the lid and bake for an additional 15-20 minutes until golden brown.

5. Kombucha Pickled Vegetables:

✓ **Ingredients:**

> ➢ 1 cup Kombucha

> ➢ 1 cup water

HOMEMADE KOMBUCHA RECIPES

- ➢ 1 tablespoon salt

- ➢ 1 tablespoon sugar

- ➢ 1 clove garlic, sliced

- ➢ 1 teaspoon whole peppercorns

- ➢ Assorted vegetables (e.g., cucumbers, carrots, radishes)

✓ **Instructions:**

- ➢ In a saucepan, combine Kombucha, water, salt, sugar, garlic, and peppercorns. Bring to a simmer until salt and sugar dissolve.

- ➢ Pack the vegetables into sterilized jars and pour the hot brine over them, leaving some space at the top.

- ➢ Seal the jars and let them cool to room temperature before refrigerating.

- ➢ Allow the vegetables to pickle for at least 24 hours before consuming.

Cooking with Kombucha opens up a world of culinary possibilities, adding unique flavors and nutritional benefits to your dishes. By incorporating this versatile ingredient into marinades, dressings, sauces, baked goods, and more, you can enhance both the taste and healthfulness of your meals. Whether you're a seasoned chef or a home cook, experimenting with Kombucha in your recipes can lead to delicious and innovative creations that go beyond the glass. Enjoy the journey of culinary exploration and the benefits of incorporating Kombucha into your diet in diverse and delightful ways.

9.2 Kombucha in Beauty and Skincare

Kombucha, known for its health benefits when consumed, also boasts numerous benefits when used in beauty and skincare routines. Its rich array of probiotics, antioxidants, and vitamins can help improve skin health, enhance the complexion, and even address specific skin concerns. This section will explore the various ways Kombucha can be incorporated into your beauty and skincare regimen, detailing its benefits, applications, and DIY recipes.

The Benefits of Kombucha for Skin

1. **Probiotics for Skin Health:**

   ✓ **Microbiome Balance:** Kombucha contains beneficial probiotics that help maintain the skin's microbiome, promoting a balanced environment that can reduce acne, inflammation, and other skin issues.

✓ **Barrier Function:** Probiotics strengthen the skin's natural barrier, protecting against environmental stressors and pollutants.

2. **Antioxidant Power:**

✓ **Free Radical Defense:** Kombucha is rich in antioxidants, such as polyphenols and vitamins C and E, which help combat free radicals, reducing oxidative stress and preventing premature aging.

✓ **Skin Repair:** Antioxidants promote cell regeneration and repair, leading to a healthier and more youthful complexion.

3. **Hydration and Brightening:**

✓ **Moisture Retention:** Kombucha helps improve the skin's moisture retention, keeping it hydrated and supple.

✓ **Brightening Effects:** The vitamins and organic acids in Kombucha can brighten the skin, reducing the appearance of dark spots and evening out skin tone.

4. **Detoxification:**

   ✓ **Cleansing:** Kombucha's detoxifying properties help cleanse the skin, removing impurities and toxins that can clog pores and cause breakouts.

Applications of Kombucha in Skincare

1. Toners:

   ✓ **Balancing Toner:** Kombucha can be used as a facial toner to balance the skin's pH, tighten pores, and prepare the skin for moisturizers and serums.

   ✓ **DIY Recipe:** Mix equal parts Kombucha and distilled water in a spray bottle. Add a few drops of essential oils like tea tree or lavender for additional benefits. Use after cleansing to tone and refresh the skin.

2. Face Masks:

   ✓ **Hydrating Mask:** Kombucha can be incorporated into face masks to deliver hydration and nutrients directly to the skin.

✓ **DIY Recipe:** Combine 2 tablespoons of Kombucha with 1 tablespoon of honey and 1 tablespoon of plain yogurt. Apply to the face, leave on for 15-20 minutes, and rinse off with warm water.

3. Exfoliants:

✓ **Gentle Exfoliation:** The natural acids in Kombucha can help exfoliate dead skin cells, promoting a smoother and more radiant complexion.

✓ **DIY Recipe:** Mix 2 tablespoons of Kombucha with 1 tablespoon of sugar and a few drops of lemon juice. Gently massage onto the skin in circular motions, then rinse with warm water.

4. Serums:

✓ **Nourishing Serum:** Kombucha can be used in serums to provide a concentrated dose of antioxidants and nutrients to the skin.

✓ **DIY Recipe:** Blend 1 tablespoon of Kombucha with 1 teaspoon of aloe vera gel and 1 teaspoon of rosehip oil. Apply a few drops to the face after toning and before moisturizing.

5. Hair Care:

- ✓ **Scalp Health:** Kombucha can improve scalp health by balancing pH, reducing dandruff, and promoting healthy hair growth.

- ✓ **DIY Recipe:** Mix 1/4 cup of Kombucha with 1/4 cup of water. Use as a final rinse after shampooing and conditioning to boost shine and scalp health.

DIY Kombucha Skincare Recipes

1. Kombucha and Green Tea Facial Toner:

- ✓ **Ingredients:**

    - ➢ 1/2 cup brewed green tea (cooled)

    - ➢ 1/2 cup Kombucha

    - ➢ 5 drops of tea tree essential oil (optional)

- ✓ **Instructions:**

1. Brew green tea and let it cool.

2. Mix green tea and Kombucha in a bottle.

3. Add tea tree essential oil for additional antibacterial benefits.

4. Apply with a cotton pad after cleansing to tone and refresh the skin.

2. Kombucha and Clay Detox Mask:

✓ **Ingredients:**

> ➢ 2 tablespoons bentonite clay

> ➢ 1 tablespoon Kombucha

> ➢ 1 tablespoon apple cider vinegar

✓ **Instructions:**

1. In a non-metal bowl, mix bentonite clay with Kombucha and apple cider vinegar to form a paste.

2. Apply to the face, avoiding the eye area.

3. Leave on for 10-15 minutes or until the mask dries.

4. Rinse off with warm water and pat dry.

3. Kombucha Hydrating Face Mist:

✓ **Ingredients:**

> ➢ 1/2 cup Kombucha

> ➢ 1/2 cup distilled water

> ➢ 1 tablespoon rose water

HOMEMADE KOMBUCHA RECIPES

> ➢ 5 drops of lavender essential oil (optional)

✓ **Instructions:**

1. Combine Kombucha, distilled water, and rose water in a spray bottle.

2. Add lavender essential oil for a soothing aroma.

3. Shake well and spritz on the face throughout the day for hydration and refreshment.

4. Kombucha Anti-Aging Serum:

✓ **Ingredients:**

> ➢ 1 tablespoon Kombucha
>
> ➢ 1 tablespoon aloe vera gel
>
> ➢ 1 teaspoon jojoba oil
>
> ➢ 5 drops of vitamin E oil

✓ **Instructions:**

1. Mix Kombucha, aloe vera gel, jojoba oil, and vitamin E oil in a small bottle.

2. Shake well to combine.

3. Apply a few drops to the face and neck after toning, gently massaging into the skin.

Commercial Kombucha Skincare Products

For those who prefer ready-made solutions, many skincare brands have started incorporating Kombucha into their products. These products range from cleansers and toners to serums and masks, offering the benefits of Kombucha in convenient, pre-formulated options. Look for reputable brands that highlight Kombucha as a key ingredient and ensure they are free from harmful additives and preservatives.

Tips for Using Kombucha in Skincare

1. **Patch Test:** Always perform a patch test when trying new skincare products or DIY recipes to ensure you do not have an allergic reaction.

2. **Freshness:** Use fresh, high-quality Kombucha for DIY skincare recipes to maximize benefits.

3. **Storage:** Store Kombucha-based skincare products in the refrigerator to prolong their shelf life and maintain potency.

4. **Consistency:** Incorporate Kombucha into your skincare routine consistently to see the best results over time.

Kombucha's rich nutritional profile and beneficial properties make it a valuable addition to any skincare routine. Whether through DIY recipes or commercial products, Kombucha can help improve skin health, enhance the complexion, and address specific skin concerns. By exploring the various ways to use Kombucha in beauty and skincare, you can enjoy the multifaceted benefits of this versatile ingredient, both inside and out.

9.3 Kombucha for Pets

Kombucha is widely recognized for its health benefits for humans, but can it also be beneficial for our furry friends? While there is limited scientific research specifically addressing the effects of Kombucha on pets, many pet owners and holistic veterinarians have explored its potential advantages. This section will delve into the possible benefits, safety considerations, and ways to incorporate Kombucha into your pet's diet and care routine.

Potential Benefits of Kombucha for Pets

1. **Probiotic Support:**

   ✓ **Gut Health:** The probiotics in Kombucha can help maintain a healthy gut flora in pets, aiding digestion and improving nutrient absorption.

✓ **Immune Function:** A balanced gut microbiome can enhance the immune system, helping pets fight off infections and illnesses.

2. **Detoxification:**

✓ **Liver Health:** Kombucha contains glucuronic acid, which supports the liver's detoxification processes, potentially aiding in the removal of toxins from your pet's body.

3. **Skin and Coat Health:**

✓ **Shiny Coat:** The antioxidants and vitamins in Kombucha can promote a healthy, shiny coat and improve overall skin condition.

✓ **Allergy Relief:** Some pet owners report reduced itching and allergy symptoms in their pets after regular Kombucha consumption.

4. **Joint and Bone Health:**

- ✓ **Glucosamine:** Kombucha naturally contains glucosamine, which can support joint health and alleviate symptoms of arthritis and joint pain in older pets.

Safety Considerations

Before introducing Kombucha to your pet's diet, it is crucial to consider safety and potential risks:

1. **Consult a Veterinarian:**

   - ✓ Always consult your veterinarian before adding any new supplement, including Kombucha, to your pet's diet. They can provide personalized advice based on your pet's health status and needs.

2. **Start Slowly:**

   - ✓ Introduce Kombucha gradually to avoid digestive upset. Start with small amounts and monitor your pet's reaction.

3. **Avoid Flavored Kombucha:**

   - ✓ Use plain, unflavored Kombucha to avoid ingredients that may be harmful to pets, such as artificial sweeteners or certain flavorings.

HOMEMADE KOMBUCHA RECIPES

4. Watch for Allergies:

- ✓ Monitor your pet for any signs of allergies or adverse reactions, such as vomiting, diarrhea, or skin irritation.

5. Limit Sugar:

- ✓ Kombucha contains sugar, which should be given in moderation to prevent weight gain and other health issues in pets.

How to Incorporate Kombucha into Your Pet's Diet

1. Direct Consumption:

- ✓ Add a small amount of plain, unflavored Kombucha to your pet's water or food. Start with a teaspoon for small pets or a tablespoon for larger pets and adjust based on their tolerance and size.

2. Kombucha Treats:

- ✓ Mix Kombucha with your pet's favorite treats. For example, you can create frozen treats by mixing Kombucha with yogurt or broth and freezing them in ice cube trays.

HOMEMADE KOMBUCHA RECIPES

3. **Topical Application:**

   ✓ For pets with skin issues, Kombucha can be applied topically. Dilute Kombucha with water (1:1 ratio) and use a spray bottle to apply it to the affected area. This can help soothe itching and irritation.

DIY Kombucha Recipes for Pets

1. Kombucha and Yogurt Frozen Treats:

   ✓ **Ingredients:**

   ➢ 1 cup plain, unflavored Kombucha

   ➢ 1 cup plain, unsweetened yogurt

   ✓ **Instructions:**

1. Mix Kombucha and yogurt in a bowl.

2. Pour the mixture into ice cube trays or silicone molds.

3. Freeze until solid.

4. Serve as a refreshing treat on hot days.

2. Kombucha Dog Biscuits:

✓ **Ingredients:**

- ➢ 1 cup whole wheat flour

- ➢ 1/2 cup rolled oats

- ➢ 1/2 cup plain, unflavored Kombucha

- ➢ 1/4 cup peanut butter (ensure it contains no xylitol)

✓ **Instructions:**

1. Preheat the oven to 350°F (175°C).

2. Mix all ingredients in a bowl to form a dough.

3. Roll out the dough on a floured surface and cut it into desired shapes.

4. Place the biscuits on a baking sheet and bake for 20-25 minutes or until golden brown.

5. Allow to cool completely before serving.

3. Kombucha for Cats:

✓ **Ingredients:**

> ➤ 1 tablespoon plain, unflavored Kombucha

> ➤ 1/2 cup tuna in water (drained)

✓ **Instructions:**

1. Mix the Kombucha with the drained tuna.

2. Serve a small portion as a treat or mix it with your cat's regular food.

Monitoring and Adjusting

1. **Observe Your Pet:**

   ✓ Keep a close eye on your pet's behavior and health after introducing Kombucha. Look for signs of improved digestion, energy levels, and coat condition.

2. **Adjust Dosage:**

   ✓ If your pet shows positive effects, you can gradually increase the amount of Kombucha. However, always stay within safe limits to avoid any potential side effects.

3. **Discontinue If Necessary:**

✓ If your pet exhibits any adverse reactions, discontinue use immediately and consult your veterinarian.

While Kombucha can offer several potential health benefits for pets, it is essential to proceed with caution and consult a veterinarian before making any dietary changes. By starting slowly and monitoring your pet's response, you can safely explore the use of Kombucha as a supplement to enhance their health and well-being. Whether used internally or topically, Kombucha can be a valuable addition to your pet care routine, promoting gut health, skin condition, and overall vitality.

9.4 Using Kombucha in the Garden

Kombucha, a fermented tea known for its probiotic benefits for humans, also has surprising uses in the garden. Its natural acidity, beneficial microbes, and nutrients can enhance soil health, support plant growth, and even deter pests. This section explores the various ways to use Kombucha in gardening, providing practical tips and DIY recipes to help you integrate this versatile beverage into your green space.

Benefits of Using Kombucha in the Garden

HOMEMADE KOMBUCHA RECIPES

1. **Soil Enrichment:**

   - ✓ **Nutrient Boost:** Kombucha contains vitamins, minerals, and organic acids that can enrich the soil, providing essential nutrients for plant growth.

   - ✓ **Microbial Activity:** The beneficial microbes in Kombucha can enhance soil microbial activity, improving soil structure and fertility.

2. **Composting:**

   - ✓ **Accelerating Composting:** Adding Kombucha to your compost pile can speed up the decomposition process, producing rich, nutrient-dense compost more quickly.

   - ✓ **Microbial Diversity:** Kombucha can introduce a diverse range of beneficial microorganisms to the compost, enhancing its quality.

3. **Plant Growth:**

   - ✓ **Root Development:** The natural acids and nutrients in Kombucha can promote healthy root development, leading to stronger and more vigorous plants.

- ✓ **Disease Resistance:** Kombucha's probiotics can help boost plants' natural defenses against diseases, reducing the need for chemical treatments.

4. **Pest Control:**

- ✓ **Natural Pesticide:** Kombucha's acidity can deter certain pests, such as aphids and mites, providing a natural alternative to chemical pesticides.

How to Use Kombucha in the Garden

1. **Soil Conditioner:**

- ✓ **Dilution:** Mix one part Kombucha with ten parts water to create a soil conditioner. This diluted solution can be used to water your plants, providing them with a gentle nutrient boost.

- ✓ **Application:** Apply the diluted Kombucha solution directly to the soil around the base of your plants every two to four weeks.

2. **Compost Activator:**

- ✓ **Direct Addition:** Pour Kombucha directly onto your compost pile to accelerate the decomposition process.

- ✓ **Dilution:** For a more controlled application, mix one part Kombucha with five parts water and sprinkle over the compost pile. Turn the compost regularly to ensure even distribution.

3. **Foliar Spray:**

- ✓ **Preparation:** Create a foliar spray by diluting Kombucha with water (1:10 ratio) and adding a few drops of mild liquid soap to help the solution adhere to the leaves.

- ✓ **Application:** Spray the diluted solution onto the leaves of your plants early in the morning or late in the evening to avoid sunburn. This can help improve nutrient uptake and deter pests.

4. **Seed Soaking:**

- ✓ **Preparation:** Soak seeds in a diluted Kombucha solution (1:10 ratio) for 24 hours before planting. This can enhance germination rates and promote strong seedling growth.

- ✓ **Application:** After soaking, plant the seeds as usual and water with a diluted Kombucha solution for the first few weeks.

5. Pest Deterrent:

- ✓ **Preparation:** Mix equal parts Kombucha and water to create a natural pest deterrent spray.

- ✓ **Application:** Spray the solution on plants affected by pests like aphids or mites. Reapply every few days until the pest problem is under control.

DIY Kombucha Gardening Recipes

1. Kombucha Plant Tonic:

- ✓ **Ingredients:**

  - ➢ 1 cup plain, unflavored Kombucha

  - ➢ 1 gallon water

HOMEMADE KOMBUCHA RECIPES

✓ **Instructions:**

1.   Mix the Kombucha and water in a large container.

2.   Use the mixture to water your plants every two to four weeks to provide a nutrient boost and enhance soil health.

2. Kombucha Compost Booster:

✓ **Ingredients:**

> ➢ 1 cup plain, unflavored Kombucha
>
> ➢ 1/2 cup molasses
>
> ➢ 5 gallons water

✓ **Instructions:**

1.   Combine Kombucha, molasses, and water in a large bucket.

2.   Stir well to dissolve the molasses.

3.   Pour the mixture over your compost pile and turn the pile to distribute evenly. Repeat every few weeks to accelerate composting.

3. Kombucha Foliar Spray:

✓ **Ingredients:**

HOMEMADE KOMBUCHA RECIPES

> ➢ 1 cup plain, unflavored Kombucha

> ➢ 10 cups water

> ➢ 1/2 teaspoon mild liquid soap

✓ **Instructions:**

1. Mix Kombucha and water in a spray bottle.

2. Add liquid soap and shake gently to combine.

3. Spray the mixture onto plant leaves early in the morning or late in the evening for best results.

4. Kombucha Seed Soak:

✓ **Ingredients:**

> ➢ 1 cup plain, unflavored Kombucha

> ➢ 10 cups water

✓ **Instructions:**

1. Mix Kombucha and water in a container.

2. Soak seeds in the solution for 24 hours before planting.

3. Plant seeds as usual and water with a diluted Kombucha solution during the initial growth phase.

5. Kombucha Pest Deterrent:

✓ **Ingredients:**

➢ 1 cup plain, unflavored Kombucha

➢ 1 cup water

✓ **Instructions:**

1. Mix Kombucha and water in a spray bottle.

2. Spray the solution directly onto affected plants, targeting areas with visible pests.

3. Reapply every few days until the pest issue is resolved.

Tips for Using Kombucha in the Garden

1. **Monitor Plant Response:**

✓ Observe how your plants respond to Kombucha applications. Adjust the concentration and frequency based on their health and growth.

2. **Avoid Overuse:**

✓ While Kombucha can be beneficial, overuse can lead to soil acidity and nutrient imbalances. Use in moderation and monitor soil pH regularly.

3. **Use Fresh Kombucha:**

✓ Ensure the Kombucha you use is fresh and free from contaminants. Avoid using flavored or sweetened Kombucha to prevent introducing harmful substances to your garden.

4. **Experiment and Adapt:**

✓ Different plants may respond differently to Kombucha. Experiment with various dilutions and application methods to find what works best for your garden.

Kombucha's natural acidity, beneficial microbes, and nutrients make it a valuable tool in gardening. By enriching the soil, boosting plant growth, and deterring pests, Kombucha can help create a healthier and more vibrant garden. Whether you're a seasoned gardener or a beginner, incorporating Kombucha into your gardening routine can offer a sustainable and eco-friendly way to enhance your plants' health and productivity.

9.5 Kombucha Crafts and DIY Projects

Kombucha isn't just a popular beverage; its versatility extends into the realm of crafts and do-it-yourself (DIY) projects. From creating unique textiles to crafting eco-friendly household items, Kombucha offers an exciting opportunity to explore sustainable creativity. This section explores various Kombucha craft ideas and DIY projects, providing inspiration and step-by-step instructions for incorporating this fermented tea into your creative pursuits.

Benefits of Using Kombucha in Crafts

1. Natural Textiles:

- ✓ **Biofilm Formation:** Kombucha produces a thin, flexible biofilm known as a SCOBY (Symbiotic Culture Of Bacteria and Yeast). This SCOBY can be used to create bio-textiles, offering a sustainable alternative to synthetic fabrics.

- ✓ **Biodegradability:** Kombucha textiles are biodegradable, reducing environmental impact compared to synthetic fibers.

2. Artistic Potential:

- ✓ **Surface Design:** Kombucha SCOBYs can be used as a canvas for artistic expression, allowing for unique textures and patterns in artworks and sculptures.
- ✓ **Dyeing:** Kombucha tea can be used as a natural dye, imparting earthy tones to fabrics and papers.

3. Eco-Friendly Materials:

- ✓ **Upcycling:** Repurposing Kombucha SCOBYs and tea waste into functional items promotes sustainability and reduces waste.

Kombucha Craft Ideas and DIY Projects

1. Kombucha SCOBY Bio-Textiles:

Materials Needed:

- ✓ Kombucha SCOBY
- ✓ Scissors
- ✓ Fabric dye (optional)

✓ Embroidery hoop (optional)

Instructions:

1. Prepare the SCOBY: Clean and dry the Kombucha SCOBY thoroughly.
2. Cutting and Shaping: Use scissors to cut the SCOBY into desired shapes and sizes.
3. Dyeing (Optional): If desired, dye the SCOBY pieces using natural fabric dye to achieve desired colors.
4. Create Art: Use SCOBY pieces for surface design, collage, or as embellishments for textile art projects. Secure SCOBY pieces onto fabric using stitching or glue.
5. Finishing Touches: Frame finished artworks in embroidery hoops for display or incorporate them into larger textile pieces.

2. Kombucha Papermaking:

Materials Needed:

✓ Kombucha tea (strained)
✓ Blender
✓ Fine mesh sieve or cheesecloth

HOMEMADE KOMBUCHA RECIPES

- ✓ Wooden frame or mold
- ✓ Felt or cloth for pressing
- ✓ Rolling pin

Instructions:

1. Prepare the Pulp: Blend Kombucha tea until smooth.
2. Forming Sheets: Pour the blended mixture into a wooden frame or mold lined with fine mesh sieve or cheesecloth.
3. Pressing: Place a piece of felt or cloth over the pulp, then press with a rolling pin to remove excess moisture and flatten the pulp.
4. Drying: Remove the pressed pulp from the frame and allow it to dry completely. Once dry, carefully peel the paper from the cloth.

3. Kombucha Candle Holders:

Materials Needed:

- ✓ Clean, dry Kombucha SCOBY
- ✓ Small glass jar or votive holder

- ✓ Tea light candle
- ✓ Scissors

Instructions:

1. Prepare the SCOBY: Cut the Kombucha SCOBY into strips or desired shapes.
2. Wrapping the Jar: Wrap the SCOBY strips around the outside of the glass jar or votive holder, ensuring they overlap slightly to create a textured effect.
3. Securing: Tuck the ends of the SCOBY strips under each other to secure them in place.
4. Insert Candle: Place a tea light candle inside the jar. Light the candle to illuminate the textured SCOBY wrap.

4. Kombucha Planters and Pot Covers:

Materials Needed:

- ✓ Kombucha SCOBY
- ✓ Scissors
- ✓ Small plant pots or containers

Instructions:

- ✓ Prepare the SCOBY: Cut the Kombucha SCOBY into strips or larger pieces, depending on the size of your plant pots.

- ✓ Wrapping: Wrap the SCOBY pieces around the outside of the plant pots or containers, covering them completely or partially.

- ✓ Securement: Tuck the ends of the SCOBY under each other or use small pins or clips to secure them in place.

- ✓ Planting: Once the SCOBY wrap is secure, place your plants or potted herbs inside the containers. Ensure the plant's root system is properly supported.

5. Kombucha Coasters:

Materials Needed:

- ✓ Clean, dry Kombucha SCOBY
- ✓ Scissors
- ✓ Pencil or marker
- ✓ Circular template (e.g., a small plate)

Instructions:

1. Prepare the SCOBY: Clean and dry the Kombucha SCOBY thoroughly.

2. Cutting: Use a pencil or marker to trace around a circular template onto the SCOBY.

3. Cut Out Shapes: Use scissors to cut out the circular shapes from the SCOBY, ensuring they are evenly shaped.

4. Drying: Allow the SCOBY coasters to dry completely on a flat surface.

5. Finishing: Once dry, use the coasters to protect surfaces from drink rings and spills. Optionally, decorate the coasters with designs or patterns using markers or dye.

Tips for Kombucha Crafts

1. **SCOBY Handling:**

   ✓ Ensure SCOBYs are clean and dry before using them in crafts to prevent mold growth and maintain quality.

2. **Experiment with Dyes:**

   ✓ Use natural fabric dyes or food-safe colors to add vibrancy to Kombucha-based crafts.

3. **Creative Expression:**

✓ Explore different techniques and applications to unleash your creativity with Kombucha crafts, from sculpture to mixed media art.

4. Educational Opportunities:

✓ Engage in educational activities by involving children or students in Kombucha crafts, teaching them about sustainability and fermentation.

Kombucha offers a wealth of creative possibilities beyond its traditional use as a beverage. By harnessing its unique properties and versatility, you can explore a range of sustainable crafts and DIY projects. Whether you're interested in textile art, papermaking, or creating functional household items, incorporating Kombucha into your crafting endeavors allows you to embrace eco-friendly practices and showcase your artistic flair. Enjoy the journey of experimentation and innovation with Kombucha crafts, transforming this fermented tea into unique and sustainable creations.

CHAPTER TEN

MAINTAINING YOUR KOMBUCHA ROUTINE

10.1 Storing and Reviving Your SCOBY

Once you've started brewing Kombucha, maintaining a healthy SCOBY (Symbiotic Culture Of Bacteria and Yeast) is essential for continuous batches of delicious, probiotic-rich tea. This section covers the best practices for storing your SCOBY between brews, reviving a dormant SCOBY, and troubleshooting common issues to ensure your Kombucha brewing routine remains successful and sustainable.

Storing Your SCOBY

1. **SCOBY Hotel:**

   ✓ **Purpose:** A SCOBY hotel is a dedicated container where you store excess SCOBYs between batches.

   ✓ **Container:** Use a large glass jar or container with enough room to hold multiple SCOBYs and enough Kombucha starter liquid to cover them completely.

- ✓ **Maintenance:** Store the SCOBY hotel in a cool, dark place, away from direct sunlight and extreme temperatures.

- ✓ **Feeding:** Check the SCOBYs monthly, discarding any that appear unhealthy or discolored. Feed the remaining SCOBYs with fresh sweet tea (regular Kombucha brew) every 2-3 months to keep them active and healthy.

2. **Refrigeration:**

- ✓ **Method:** For longer storage, SCOBYs can be refrigerated. Place the SCOBY in a glass container filled with Kombucha starter liquid (plain Kombucha from a recent batch).

- ✓ **Duration:** SCOBYs can stay refrigerated for several weeks to a few months without significant loss of viability.

- ✓ **Revival:** Before using a refrigerated SCOBY for brewing, allow it to come to room temperature. Feed it with fresh sweet tea and wait until it shows signs of fermentation activity (formation of a new layer or bubbles).

Reviving a Dormant SCOBY

1. **Room Temperature Revival:**

   ✓ **Process:** Take the SCOBY out of storage and let it come to room temperature. Place it in a clean glass container and add fresh sweet tea (cooled brewed tea with sugar dissolved in it).

   ✓ **Observation:** Watch for signs of fermentation activity, such as bubbles forming and a new SCOBY layer developing at the surface.

   ✓ **Patience:** It may take several days for the SCOBY to fully revive and become active again. Be patient and allow it time to acclimate to the new brew.

2. **Troubleshooting Dormant SCOBY:**

   ✓ **No Activity:** If the SCOBY shows no signs of activity after several days, it may be too weak or contaminated. In this case, it's advisable to start fresh with a new SCOBY.

✓ **Mold:** Discard any SCOBY showing signs of mold growth. Moldy SCOBYs cannot be salvaged and should not be used for brewing.

Common Issues and Troubleshooting

1. **SCOBY Health Check:**

   ✓ **Signs of Health:** A healthy SCOBY is creamy white or beige in color, with a smooth texture and no foul odor.

   ✓ **Signs of Concern:** Discoloration (brown or black spots), a strong vinegar smell, or unusual growth patterns may indicate contamination or improper brewing conditions.

2. **Maintaining Hygiene:**

   ✓ **Clean Equipment:** Use clean, non-metallic equipment and containers for brewing and storing SCOBYs. Wash hands thoroughly before handling SCOBYs or brewing equipment to prevent contamination.

3. **Temperature and Light Control:**

   - ✓ **Ideal Conditions:** Keep brewing vessels away from direct sunlight and maintain a stable temperature between 68-78°F (20-25°C).

   - ✓ **Extreme Temperatures:** Avoid exposing SCOBYs to extreme heat or cold, as it can affect fermentation and SCOBY health.

4. **Feeding Schedule:**

   - ✓ **Regular Feeding:** SCOBYs need a constant supply of fresh sweet tea (black or green tea brewed with sugar) to thrive. Feed SCOBYs every 2-3 months in a SCOBY hotel or when reviving from storage.

Maintaining your Kombucha brewing routine revolves around proper storage and care of your SCOBY. By establishing a SCOBY hotel for storage, knowing how to revive a dormant SCOBY, and troubleshooting common issues, you can ensure consistent and successful batches of Kombucha tea. With attention to hygiene, temperature control, and regular feeding, you'll enjoy the benefits of homemade Kombucha while prolonging the lifespan and vitality of your SCOBY cultures. Embrace the art and science of Kombucha brewing, making it a rewarding and sustainable part of your culinary and wellness practices.

10.2 Scaling Up Your Brew

As your confidence and interest in brewing Kombucha grow, you may find yourself wanting to produce larger batches or experiment with different flavors and techniques. Scaling up your Kombucha brewing process requires careful planning, additional equipment, and attention to maintaining quality and consistency. This section explores how to effectively scale up your Kombucha production while ensuring successful outcomes and enjoyable brewing experiences.

Considerations for Scaling Up

1. **Equipment Upgrade:**

   ✓ **Large Brewing Vessel:** Invest in a larger glass brewing vessel or food-grade plastic fermenter that can accommodate the increased volume of tea and SCOBY.

✓ **Airlocks and Covers:** Ensure your vessel has a tight-fitting lid with an airlock to maintain proper fermentation conditions and prevent contamination.

2. **Ingredients Quantity:**

✓ **Tea and Sugar:** Increase the amount of tea leaves and sugar proportionally to the batch size. Use high-quality black or green tea without additives for consistent flavor and SCOBY health.

✓ **Starter Liquid:** Maintain the ratio of starter liquid (previously brewed Kombucha) to fresh sweet tea to ensure a healthy fermentation process.

3. **Temperature Control:**

✓ **Consistent Environment:** Maintain a stable brewing temperature between 68-78°F (20-25°C). Consider using a temperature-controlled fermentation chamber or a dedicated space away from drafts and direct sunlight.

4. **Brewing Schedule:**

   ✓ **Batch Timing:** Plan your brewing schedule to accommodate the longer fermentation times required for larger batches. Monitor the fermentation progress regularly to ensure the desired level of tartness and flavor development.

5. **Sanitation and Hygiene:**

   ✓ **Cleanliness:** Scale up your sanitization practices to prevent contamination. Use non-metallic utensils and thoroughly clean all equipment before and after use.

Steps to Scale Up Your Kombucha Brew

1. **Calculate Batch Size:**

   ✓ **Volume Calculation:** Determine the desired batch size based on your brewing vessel's capacity and available storage space. Consider starting with a manageable increase, such as doubling or tripling your current batch size.

HOMEMADE KOMBUCHA RECIPES

2. **Prepare Equipment:**

   ✓ **Upgrade Equipment:** Acquire larger brewing vessels, fermentation locks, and storage containers. Ensure all equipment is food-grade and suitable for prolonged contact with Kombucha.

3. **Adjust Recipe Proportions:**

   ✓ **Ingredient Scaling:** Scale up the amount of tea leaves, sugar, and starter liquid proportionally to the batch size. Maintain the standard ratio of 1 cup of sugar and 8 tea bags (or equivalent) per gallon of water.

4. **Monitor Fermentation:**

   ✓ **Observation:** During fermentation, monitor the pH level and taste of the Kombucha regularly. Adjust fermentation times or conditions as needed to achieve the desired flavor profile and acidity level.

5. **Storage and Bottling:**

✓ **Container Options:** Transfer the fermented Kombucha to clean glass bottles or jars for secondary fermentation or storage. Ensure containers are sealed tightly to promote carbonation and flavor development.

6. **Flavoring and Experimentation:**

✓ **Creative Freedom:** With larger batches, experiment with different flavor combinations, herbs, fruits, or spices during secondary fermentation. Maintain careful notes to replicate successful recipes in future batches.

Scaling Up Tips

✓ **Gradual Expansion:** Start with a modest increase in batch size to familiarize yourself with the process and ensure consistent results.

✓ **Record Keeping:** Maintain detailed records of ingredients, brewing times, and flavor experiments to refine your brewing techniques and troubleshoot issues.

✓ **Community and Resources:** Join online forums, local clubs, or workshops to exchange tips and experiences with other Kombucha enthusiasts scaling up their brewing operations.

Scaling up your Kombucha brewing operation allows you to explore new flavors, share your creations with friends and family, and potentially turn your hobby into a rewarding culinary endeavor. By investing in larger equipment, maintaining meticulous sanitation practices, and adhering to a disciplined brewing schedule, you can confidently produce quality batches of Kombucha tea. Embrace the journey of scaling up your brew, experimenting with flavors, and refining your techniques to enjoy the health benefits and delicious taste of homemade Kombucha on a larger scale.

10.3 Sharing and Gifting Kombucha

Sharing homemade Kombucha is a delightful way to introduce others to the benefits and flavors of this probiotic-rich beverage. Whether you're brewing for friends, family, or special occasions, this section explores the art of sharing and gifting Kombucha, including packaging ideas, safety considerations, and tips for ensuring your brews are well-received and appreciated.

Benefits of Sharing Kombucha

1. **Health Benefits:** Introducing others to the health benefits of Kombucha, such as improved digestion, boosted immunity, and overall wellness.

2. **Culinary Experience:** Sharing unique flavors and creative recipes with friends and family, showcasing your brewing skills and creativity.

3. **Community Building:** Building connections and community through shared experiences and discussions about fermentation and wellness.

Tips for Sharing Kombucha

1. **Packaging and Presentation:**

   ✓ **Clean Bottles:** Use clean, sanitized glass bottles with secure closures (such as swing-top lids) to ensure freshness and prevent carbonation loss.

   ✓ **Labeling:** Label each bottle with the flavor and brewing date. Include any special ingredients or brewing notes for recipients to enjoy and appreciate.

   ✓ **Gift Packaging:** Consider presenting Kombucha bottles in a decorative box or basket, along with information about Kombucha and its health benefits.

2. **Safety and Hygiene:**

   ✓ **Sanitation:** Maintain strict sanitation practices throughout the brewing, bottling, and gifting process to prevent contamination.

   ✓ **Storage Conditions:** Store bottled Kombucha in a cool, dark place away from direct sunlight to preserve flavor and carbonation.

3. **Educational Resources:**

   ✓ **Information Sheets:** Include informational sheets or recipes with each gift to educate recipients about Kombucha and how to enjoy it safely.

Gifting Kombucha Ideas

1. **Holiday and Special Occasions:**

✓ **Custom Flavors:** Create seasonal flavors (e.g., cranberry-orange for winter holidays) to gift during festive occasions.

✓ **Gift Sets:** Prepare gift sets with multiple flavors or include homemade Kombucha accessories, such as SCOBYs or brewing kits.

2. **Weddings and Celebrations:**

✓ **Personalized Labels:** Customize labels with the couple's names and wedding date for a memorable and health-conscious wedding favor.

✓ **Toast Alternative:** Offer Kombucha as a non-alcoholic option for toasts and celebrations, catering to health-conscious guests.

3. **Workplace and Corporate Gifts:**

✓ **Health and Wellness:** Promote wellness in the workplace by gifting Kombucha as a refreshing and beneficial beverage option.

✓ **Teambuilding:** Use Kombucha brewing workshops or tastings as team-building activities, fostering camaraderie and healthy habits among colleagues.

Etiquette and Considerations

1. **Recipient Preferences:**

   ✓ **Allergies and Preferences:** Consider dietary restrictions, allergies, and preferences (e.g., low sugar) when selecting flavors or brewing styles for gifts.

   ✓ **Introduction:** Introduce newcomers to Kombucha gradually, starting with milder flavors or lower carbonation levels.

2. **Legal and Safety Considerations:**

   ✓ **Labeling Requirements:** Ensure compliance with local regulations regarding homemade food and beverage gifts, including labeling and distribution guidelines.

✓ **Responsibility:** Inform recipients about the fermentation process and any potential risks associated with consuming homemade Kombucha.

Sharing and gifting Kombucha is a rewarding way to spread joy, wellness, and culinary creativity with others. By following best practices for packaging, safety, and consideration of recipient preferences, you can confidently share your homemade brews and introduce others to the delightful world of Kombucha. Whether for holidays, special occasions, or everyday enjoyment, gifting Kombucha fosters connections, promotes wellness, and celebrates the art of homemade fermentation. Embrace the opportunity to share your passion for Kombucha brewing, leaving a flavorful and healthful impression on those around you.

CONCLUSION

In conclusion, this guidebook has explored the multifaceted world of Kombucha, offering a comprehensive journey from its origins and health benefits to practical brewing techniques and creative recipes. Whether you're a beginner eager to embark on your first batch of Kombucha or a senior looking to adapt recipes to suit your dietary needs, this guidebook has provided the tools, knowledge, and inspiration to embark on a fulfilling Kombucha brewing experience.

For beginners, we've covered the essentials: understanding SCOBY, selecting ingredients, mastering fermentation, and troubleshooting common issues. Detailed step-by-step recipes, from classic brews to vibrant flavor combinations, have empowered you to experiment and create Kombucha tailored to your taste.

For seniors, specialized chapters have addressed low-sugar options, gentle flavors, and nutrient-boosted recipes, ensuring that Kombucha can be enjoyed as a part of a balanced diet and wellness routine.

Beyond the brewing process, this guidebook has explored the versatility of Kombucha, from its potential in cooking and skincare to its use in crafting and gardening. It has highlighted the role of Kombucha in promoting digestive health, boosting immunity, and supporting detoxification, underlining its holistic benefits beyond mere refreshment.

HOMEMADE KOMBUCHA RECIPES

Moreover, we've delved into the joys of sharing Kombucha with others, from gifting personalized brews to fostering community through homemade wellness initiatives.

Whether you're intrigued by the science of fermentation or captivated by the creative possibilities of flavoring and crafting, Kombucha offers a journey of exploration and enjoyment. As you continue on your Kombucha brewing adventure, remember to embrace experimentation, cherish the process, and share your passion with others. May your cups be filled with health, flavor, and the satisfaction of homemade goodness. Cheers to your continued success and enjoyment with Kombucha!

THANKS FOR YOUR ATTENTION!!!

www.ingramcontent.com/pod-product-compliance
Lightning Source LLC
Chambersburg PA
CBHW051550250726

48653CB00004BA/1079